MRCP
PAEDIATRIC
MCQS WITH INDIVIDUAL
SUBJECT SUMMARIES

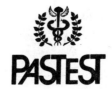

PASTEST

MRCP PART 1 PAEDIATRIC MCQS WITH INDIVIDUAL SUBJECT SUMMARIES

Dr R M Beattie
Consultant Paediatrician,
Peterborough District Hospital

© 1997 PASTEST
Egerton Court
Parkgate Estate
Knutsford
Cheshire WA16 8DX

First published 1997
Reprinted 1998

ISBN 0 906896 74 6

A catalogue record for this book is available from the British Library.

Text prepared by Breeze Ltd, Manchester
Printed by Athenæum Press Ltd, Gateshead, Tyne & Wear

CONTENTS

CONTRIBUTORS

Dr R M Beattie, Consultant Paediatrician

Dr A B Acharya, Senior Registrar

Dr D L I Ellis, Senior House Officer

Dr A T Tidswell, Senior House Officer

Department of Paediatrics
Peterborough District Hospital
Thorpe Road
Peterborough
PE3 6DA

INTRODUCTION

The MRCP Part 1 examination is a major hurdle for the aspiring paediatrician. To pass requires a thorough knowledge of applied basic science, paediatrics and general medicine. This is an awesome proposition for most junior doctors. This book is designed to help.

The MCQs in this book have been written in the style of the examination and cover many frequently asked topics. The subject summaries provide carefully structured and highly relevant teaching material and also highlight other potential MCQ stems.

I have prepared this book with assistance from a number of people who have recently taken the exam. We hope that exam candidates will find the information we have compiled helpful. A bibliography is included for further reading and as a reference source for the information quoted.

I would like to acknowledge the following people who have read and commented on various sections of the book as they were written - Dr Iolanda Guarino, Dr L Ng, Dr W Hyer, Dr Anne Smith, Dr K N Chan, Dr D M Johnston and Dr J A Kuzemo. I would also like to acknowledge the enthusiasm and hard work of Dr T Tidswell, Dr D Ellis and Dr A B Acharya who produced numerous questions and well-researched explanations for the book. I would also like to thank my wife and children without whose support this book would never have materialised.

R M Beattie

PASTEST PAEDIATRIC BOOKS FOR MRCP PART 1

MRCP Part 1 Paediatric MCQ Practice Exams
Ian Maconochie MRCP   ISBN 0 906896 59 2
- Six complete MCQ papers with an authentic combination of paediatrics, general medicine and basic sciences
- Correct answers and detailed teaching notes
- Advice on MCQ exam technique
- Comprehensive index plus MCQ subject listings

MRCP Part 1 Paediatric MCQ Revision Book
Ian Maconochie MRCP Jo Wilmshurst MRCP   ISBN 0 906896 39 8
- 300 MCQs arranged by subject which are based on the new MRCP Part 1 Paediatric syllabus
- Answers and extended teaching explanations
- Comprehensive revision index
- One complete Practice Examination of 60 MCQs
This combination of subject-based MCQs and a complete practice paper will make this book invaluable to all candidates.

MRCP Part 1 Paediatric Past Topics: A Revision Syllabus
David Goldblatt MRCP PhD   ISBN 1 901198 00 6
- Exam topics listed in order of appearance by date
- League tables indicating frequency of appearance of each topic
- Revision checklists for every subject
- Complete MCQ practice paper of 60 questions with teaching notes
This book has been written in response to demand from doctors and is an invaluable material for doctors planning their revision.

Explanations to the Royal College Red Booklet
ISBN 0 906896 54 1 *available by mail order only*
- Answers and expert teaching notes related to the RCP red book of sample paediatric exam questions
- Emphasis on favourite Membership papers
Indispensable insight and guidance for all MRCP Part 1 paediatric candidates.

For full details of the range of PasTest books and courses available for MRCP Part 1 candidates, contact PasTest today:

PasTest, Egerton Court, Parkgate Estate,
Knutsford, Cheshire WA16 8DX
Telephone 01565 755226 Fax 01565 650264

CARDIOLOGY

1. In the neonate presenting with central cyanosis

☐ A   the hyperoxia test is used to confirm patency of the ductus arteriosus
☐ B   acrocyanosis is indicative of central cyanosis
☐ C   a physiological right to left shunt must be present
☐ D   more than 5 g/dl of haemoglobin is in the reduced state
☐ E   prostaglandin therapy may be appropriate

2. In Down's syndrome

☐ A   the commonest cardiac lesion is an atrial septal defect
☐ B   echocardiography is indicated even if a murmur is not present
☐ C   20% have associated heart defects
☐ D   tetralogy of Fallot is a recognised association
☐ E   the cardiac defects are the sole cause of pulmonary vascular disease

3. Transposition of the great arteries

☐ A   is associated with increased pulmonary blood flow
☐ B   is the commonest cause of cyanotic congenital heart disease in the neonatal period
☐ C   is associated with a metabolic alkalosis
☐ D   can be corrected by the Jatene (arterial switch) procedure
☐ E   has atrioventricular block as a recognised complication

4. In tetralogy of Fallot

☐ A   the murmur becomes louder during cyanotic spells
☐ B   polycythaemia is a recognised finding
☐ C   an atrial septal defect is a component of the tetralogy
☐ D   clubbing develops within the first 3 months
☐ E   right ventricular hypertrophy is present

5. **Which of the following conditions can present in the neonatal period with central cyanosis:**

☐   A   Eisenmenger's syndrome
☐   B   pulmonary atresia
☐   C   hypoplastic left heart
☐   D   transposition of the great arteries
☐   E   aortic stenosis

6. **Regarding the paediatric ECG**

☐   A   neonates have right axis deviation
☐   B   complete heart block is associated with maternal systemic lupus erythematosus
☐   C   right bundle branch block is seen in coarctation of the aorta
☐   D   Romano Ward syndrome produces prolongation of the PR interval
☐   E   a resting heart rate in newborns of 180 is a tachycardia

7. **Which of the following chest X-ray findings would support the paired diagnosis:**

☐   A   atrio septal defect and coeur en sabot (heart in a boot)
☐   B   patent ductus arteriosus and rib notching
☐   C   truncus arteriosus and absent thymus
☐   D   total anomalous pulmonaryvenous drainage and cottage loaf appearance
☐   E   scimitar syndrome and dextrocardia

8. **Which of the following conditions are associated with an increased incidence of heart disease:**

☐   A   Kawasaki's disease
☐   B   congenital rubella
☐   C   Marfan's syndrome
☐   D   Turner's syndrome
☐   E   petit mal epilepsy

9. Which of the following statements are true:

☐ A the commonest congenital cardiac lesion is an atrioventricular septal defect

☐ B tetralogy of Fallot is associated with plethoric lung fields

☐ C the Blalock-Taussig shunt gives rise to a continuous murmur

☐ D nitrous oxide can be used to treat persistent pulmonary hypertension

☐ E Ebstein's anomaly is an anomaly of the tricuspid valve

10. Which of the following statements concerning atrial septal defects are correct:

☐ A ostium secundum defects are commoner then ostium primum defects

☐ B atrial fibrillation is a recognised associated complication

☐ C in a secundum defect the ECG shows right bundle branch block and left axis deviation

☐ D the pulmonary vascular resistance increases in early childhood

☐ E a left to right shunt of more than 2:1 is an indication for surgical closure

11. Ventricular septal defects

☐ A are usually located in the muscular part of the ventricular septum

☐ B in the neonate will always cause a flow murmur across the defect which is present from birth

☐ C infective endocarditis is a complication in 10%

☐ D are associated with a higher oxygen content in the blood of the right ventricle than the right atrium

☐ E are associated with right ventricular volume overload

12. Eisenmenger's syndrome can result from:

☐ A pulmonary artery stenosis

☐ B total anomalous pulmonary venous drainage

☐ C tetralogy of Fallot

☐ D aortopulmonary window

☐ E ventricular septal defect

13. Patent ductus arteriosus

- [ ] A is commoner in females
- [ ] B is commoner in preterm infants
- [ ] C can be treated with prostaglandins
- [ ] D usually closes spontaneously in term infants
- [ ] E may present as recurrent apnoea

14. Concerning the fetal circulation

- [ ] A the umbilical vein carries deoxygenated blood to the placenta from the fetus
- [ ] B fetal superior vena caval blood preferentially flows across the foramen ovale into the left atrium
- [ ] C 40% of right ventricular outflow enters the lungs
- [ ] D the descending aorta is connected to the pulmonary artery via the ductus venosus
- [ ] E gas exchange occurs in the fetal lungs

15. Which of the following statements are true:

- [ ] A patients with cyanotic congenital heart disease grow normally
- [ ] B immunisation is contraindicated in children with congenital heart disease
- [ ] C the oral contraceptive pill is contraindicated in patients with prosthetic heart valves
- [ ] D 2% of patients with congenital heart disease have a chromosomal abnormality
- [ ] E 30% of infants with chromosomal defects have heart defects

16. Coarctation of the aorta

- [ ] A is associated with bicuspid aortic valves
- [ ] B is associated with rib notching in infancy
- [ ] C is a feature of Edward's syndrome
- [ ] D is more common in females
- [ ] E may be associated with blood pressure discrepancy in the upper limbs

17. Which of the following cardiac defects and teratogens are correctly paired:

☐ A alcohol and transposition of the great arteries
☐ B sodium valproate and aortic stenosis
☐ C frusemide and patent ductus arteriosus
☐ D phenytoin and coarctation of the aorta
☐ E lithium and Ebstein's anomaly

18. In childhood hypertension

☐ A systolic pressure greater than the 75th centile for age and gender is the correct definition
☐ B primary is more common than secondary hypertension
☐ C irrespective of age the commonest cause is renal artery stenosis
☐ D children with primary hypertension are usually symptomatic
☐ E there is little point in obtaining blood or urine for analysis

19. Which of the following are causes of circulatory failure in the first week of life:

☐ A arrhythmias
☐ B hypoplastic left heart
☐ C birth asphyxia
☐ D severe anaemia
☐ E fluid overload

20. Concerning infective endocarditis

☐ A *E. coli* is the commonest cause
☐ B antibiotic prophylaxis is indicated to cover dental procedures in a child with an ostium secundum atrial septal defect
☐ C splinter haemorrhages in the nail beds are an almost universal finding
☐ D the diagnosis is excluded if echocardiography is normal
☐ E it is usually the right side of the heart that is affected

21. Which of the following are correct:

- [ ] A hypertrophic obstructive cardiomyopathy can be inherited as an autosomal dominant
- [ ] B dilated cardiomyopathy is associated with adriamycin toxicity in children
- [ ] C restrictive cardiomyopathy is the commonest cardiomyopathy in childhood
- [ ] D endocardial fibroelastosis is a form of hypertrophic cardiomyopathy
- [ ] E there is an increased incidence of dilated cardiomyopathy in infants of diabetic mothers

22. Rheumatic fever

- [ ] A occurs secondary to infection with beta-haemolytic *Streptococcus* group A
- [ ] B causes a pancarditis
- [ ] C is associated with upper socio-economic class
- [ ] D PR prolongation on the ECG is one of the major diagnostic criteria
- [ ] E prophylactic antibiotics should be stopped after 3 months

23. The following support the diagnosis of an innocent murmur:

- [ ] A present only in diastole
- [ ] B fixed splitting of S2
- [ ] C heard only in high output states
- [ ] D heard all over the praecordium
- [ ] E variable with position and posture

24. Cardiac emergencies

- [ ] A asynchronous DC shock is the appropriate treatment for a supraventricular tachycardia
- [ ] B DC shock is the appropriate treatment of electromechanical dissociation
- [ ] C atropine is the first-line drug for asystole
- [ ] D ventricular fibrillation is a common cardiac arrhythmia in childhood
- [ ] E lignocaine may be given via an intraosseus needle

25. Which of the following are true:

☐   A   head injury can cause prolongation of the QT interval
☐   B   the normal PR interval in infancy is 0.2–0.3 s
☐   C   myxomas are the commonest cardiac tumours in childhood
☐   D   cerebral abscess is a rare complication of congenital heart disease under the age of 2 years
☐   E   a third heart sound can be normal in childhood

26. Lymphocytic interstitial pneumonitis

- ☐ A has an insidious onset in most cases
- ☐ B usually presents in the first year of life
- ☐ C has a mortality greater than 50%
- ☐ D is due to *Pneumocystis carinii* infection
- ☐ E responds to oral steroids

27. The clearance of theophylline is increased by

- ☐ A cirrhosis
- ☐ B fever
- ☐ C phenytoin
- ☐ D cigarette smoking
- ☐ E erythromycin

28. *Pneumocystis carinii* pneumonia

- ☐ A is a viral infection
- ☐ B rarely presents under the age of one
- ☐ C can be treated with high dose penicillin
- ☐ D has a high mortality
- ☐ E can be present with a normal chest X-ray

29. Signs of acute severe asthma include

- ☐ A pulsus paradoxus > 20 mmHg
- ☐ B cyanosis
- ☐ C intercostal recession
- ☐ D hyperexpanded chest
- ☐ E pyrexia

30. Pulmonary hypoplasia in the newborn

- ☐ A can be idiopathic
- ☐ B is associated with oligohydramnios
- ☐ C is seen in 1 in 10 000 births
- ☐ D can be unilateral
- ☐ E occurs in Potter's syndrome

31. Concerning acute stridor in childhood

- ☐ A the most common cause is acute laryngotracheobronchitis
- ☐ B acute epiglottitis is a rare cause
- ☐ C antibiotics should be given if the diagnosis is acute laryngotracheobronchitis
- ☐ D steroids are helpful if bacterial tracheitis is the diagnosis
- ☐ E nebulised adrenaline can be used even if the diagnosis is not known

32. Concerning bronchiolitis

- ☐ A most cases are in children under 6 months
- ☐ B 25% of cases are due to respiratory syncitial virus
- ☐ C antibiotics are indicated in all children under 3 months at presentation
- ☐ D nebulised ipratropium bromide is often beneficial
- ☐ E steroids are unhelpful

33. The following are characteristic of type II respiratory failure:

- ☐ A hyperventilation
- ☐ B hypoxia
- ☐ C ventilation perfusion mismatch
- ☐ D raised $PaCO_2$
- ☐ E head injury as a possible cause

34. Concerning laryngomalacia

☐ A   it is the most common cause of persistent stridor in infancy
☐ B   prognosis is poor
☐ C   it is rarely present at birth
☐ D   failure to thrive is a common manifestation
☐ E   laryngoscopy is indicated in all cases

35. Useful agents taken immediately before exercise in order to prevent exercise-induced asthma include

☐ A   sodium cromoglycate
☐ B   salbutamol
☐ C   fluticasone propionate
☐ D   terbutaline
☐ E   salmeterol

36. Rigid bronchoscopy is generally required

☐ A   to remove a foreign body
☐ B   to exclude a vocal cord palsy
☐ C   to diagnose tuberculosis
☐ D   to assess persistent atelectasis
☐ E   to remove a blood clot

37. Causes of a false-positive sweat test include

☐ A   ventricular septal defect
☐ B   adrenal insufficiency
☐ C   pseudohypoaldosteronism
☐ D   asthma
☐ E   chronic renal failure

38. In children with cleft lip and palate the following are true:

☐ A   it is an abnormality of mesodermal development
☐ B   there are associated abnormalities in more than 75%
☐ C   micrognathia is common
☐ D   recurrence risk in siblings is 1 in 25
☐ E   grommets are usually required

39. Which of the following suggest epiglottitis rather than viral croup:

☐ A   short history
☐ B   pyrexia
☐ C   good response to nebulised adrenaline
☐ D   neck extension
☐ E   toxaemia

40. The following methods of administration of beta agonists are appropriate in a four year old with chronic asthma:

☐ A   nebuliser
☐ B   inhaler with a spacer device
☐ C   turbohaler
☐ D   dischaler
☐ E   oral medication

41. Primary ciliary dyskinesia

☐ A   is an autosomally recessively inherited group of disorders
☐ B   males are usually infertile
☐ C   is a cause of conductive hearing loss
☐ D   is associated with situs inversus in 75%
☐ E   normal life expectancy is possible

42. Concerning cystic fibrosis

- ☐ A clubbing is a feature
- ☐ B inheritance is autosomal recessive
- ☐ C the gene is on chromosome 6
- ☐ D males are almost universally infertile
- ☐ E meconium ileus is the presenting feature in 50%

43. Causes of bronchiectasis include

- ☐ A cirrhosis
- ☐ B asthma
- ☐ C foreign body
- ☐ D cystic fibrosis
- ☐ E pneumococcal infection

44. Obstructive sleep apnoea

- ☐ A is an indication for adenotonsillectomy
- ☐ B results in episodes of hypoxia
- ☐ C is a cause of daytime sleepiness
- ☐ D causes left ventricular hypertrophy
- ☐ E can present with hypercapnia

45. In *Mycoplasma pneumoniae* infection

- ☐ A the infection is spread by droplets
- ☐ B erythromycin is the drug of choice
- ☐ C cold agglutinins are present in 50%
- ☐ D culture is easily obtained
- ☐ E headache at presentation is unusual

46. Which of the following statements are true concerning tonsillitis:

- ☐ A bacterial is commoner than viral infection
- ☐ B pus on the tonsils is diagnostic of bacterial infection
- ☐ C agranulocytosis is a recognised differential diagnosis
- ☐ D post-operative bleeding should be managed with local pressure
- ☐ E quinsy is an indication for tonsillectomy

47. The following are appropriate in the immediate management of anaphylactic shock:

- ☐ A oral chlorpheniramine maleate
- ☐ B i.v. hydrocortisone
- ☐ C nebulised salbutamol
- ☐ D i.v. adrenaline
- ☐ E endotracheal adrenaline

48. Concerning pulmonary tuberculosis

- ☐ A *Mycobacterium tuberculosis* is commonly found in the soil
- ☐ B it is a notifiable disease
- ☐ C pleural effusions may occur
- ☐ D most children develop cavitating lung disease
- ☐ E a positive Mantoux test is diagnostic of infection with *Mycobacterium tuberculosis*

49. Which of the following are present in the lung in their adult quota at birth:

- ☐ A alveoli
- ☐ B goblet cells
- ☐ C terminal bronchioles
- ☐ D pulmonary vessels
- ☐ E acini

50. The peak expiratory flow rate

☐ A is increased in obstructive airways disease
☐ B is effort independent
☐ C is a suitable measurement to attempt on a three year old
☐ D is diagnostic of asthma if the value increases by 20% after
administration of bronchodilators
☐ E is influenced by airway diameter

51. The following milks are protein hydrolysates:

- [ ] A Nutramigen
- [ ] B Prematil
- [ ] C Maxijul
- [ ] D Flexical
- [ ] E Paediasure

52. Meckel's diverticulum

- [ ] A is a remnant of the vitello-intestinal duct
- [ ] B can contain ectopic pancreatic tissue
- [ ] C is located within the jejunum
- [ ] D can present with massive blood loss per rectum
- [ ] E is a cause of intussusception

53. Absolute contraindications to breast feeding include

- [ ] A infants with galactosaemia
- [ ] B maternal tuberculosis
- [ ] C maternal HIV
- [ ] D atenolol
- [ ] E cytotoxic drugs

54. Recognised consequences of abetalipoproteinaemia include

- [ ] A failure to thrive
- [ ] B autosomal dominant inheritance
- [ ] C ataxia secondary to vitamin D deficiency
- [ ] D child is normal at birth
- [ ] E retinitis pigmentosa

55. Characteristic features of acrodermatitis enteropathica include

☐ A malabsorption of copper
☐ B autosomal dominant inheritance
☐ C recurrent infections
☐ D alopecia
☐ E rapid response to treatment with zinc sulphate

56. Vitamin A

☐ A deficiency is the commonest cause of visual loss worldwide
☐ B is fat soluble
☐ C has an important role to play in resistance to infection
☐ D is present in milk
☐ E is beneficial in the management of severe measles

57. Breast feeding reduces the incidence of

☐ A atopy in infants born to mothers with a history of atopy
☐ B gastrointestinal infection
☐ C nappy rash
☐ D respiratory infection
☐ E infantile colic

58. Concerning vitamin K

☐ A in the new-born period an oral dose is as effective as an intramuscular dose in all babies
☐ B there is an association between intramuscular vitamin K and childhood cancer
☐ C it is a fat soluble vitamin
☐ D 1 mg of vitamin K i.m. ensures adequate prophylaxis in term infants
☐ E liver is a good dietary source

59. The xylose absorption test

- [ ] A   is a reliable test in children
- [ ] B   is likely to be normal in cystic fibrosis
- [ ] C   is dependent on the surface area of the small intestine
- [ ] D   is abnormal in coeliac disease
- [ ] E   requires a blood test

60. Serum folate levels are likely to be

- [ ] A   reduced in gluten-sensitive enteropathy
- [ ] B   reduced following resection of the terminal ileum
- [ ] C   reduced on treatment with anticonvulsants
- [ ] D   low in pernicious anaemia
- [ ] E   reduced as part of the acute phase response

61. The content of human milk at term per 100 ml is as follows:

- [ ] A   50 kcal
- [ ] B   1.3 g protein
- [ ] C   0.65 mmol sodium
- [ ] D   4.2 g fat
- [ ] E   7 g carbohydrate

62. Features of carbohydrate intolerance include

- [ ] A   usually inherited
- [ ] B   characterised by explosive stools
- [ ] C   usually transient
- [ ] D   reducing substances in the stool are negative
- [ ] E   commonly follows *Salmonella* infection

63. Preterm compared with term formula

- ☐ A contains more kcal per ml
- ☐ B has a lower sodium content
- ☐ C contains more calcium
- ☐ D contains more iron
- ☐ E has the same protein content

64. Human (breast) milk compared with unmodified cows' milk contains more

- ☐ A protein
- ☐ B sodium
- ☐ C calories per 100 ml
- ☐ D fat
- ☐ E calcium

65. The following statements are true of nutritional supplements:

- ☐ A Maxijul is a glucose polymer
- ☐ B Caloreen is a fat emulsion
- ☐ C Duocal contains carbohydrate and protein
- ☐ D Calogen contains 450 kcal per 100 g
- ☐ E whey based infant formulae contain more calories than casein based infant formulae

66. Immunoglobulin A

- ☐ A makes up 50% of serum immunoglobulins
- ☐ B predominates on respiratory and gastrointestinal surfaces in its secretory form
- ☐ C selective deficiency is rare with a prevalence of less than 1 in 10,000
- ☐ D deficiency is associated with an increased risk of infection
- ☐ E deficiency is associated with an increased risk of atopic disease

67. Causes of failure to thrive include

☐ A low birth weight
☐ B Duchenne muscular dystrophy
☐ C inadequate intake
☐ D renal tubular acidosis
☐ E preterm gestation

68. The following statements are true:

☐ A starch is a glucose polymer
☐ B lactose is a disaccharide made up of galactose and glucose
☐ C carbohydrate digestion is dependent on pancreatic secretion
☐ D sucrase hydrolyses sucrose into glucose and fructose
☐ E glucose, galactose and fructose are all absorbed by an active transport mechanism

69. The following are characteristic features of Wilson's disease:

☐ A low serum copper
☐ B low serum caeruloplasmin
☐ C poor response to copper chelation
☐ D Kayser-Fleischer rings
☐ E autosomal recessive inheritance

70. The following cause predominantly unconjugated hyperbilirubinaemia in the neonate:

☐ A gallstones
☐ B pyloric stenosis
☐ C ABO incompatibility
☐ D biliary atresia
☐ E glucose 6 phosphate dehydrogenase deficiency

71. Causes of a flat jejunal biopsy include

- ☐ A coeliac disease
- ☐ B glucose–galactose malabsorption
- ☐ C giardiasis
- ☐ D cystic fibrosis
- ☐ E cows' milk allergy

72. Hepatitis B

- ☐ A is a DNA virus
- ☐ B transmission is faeco-oral
- ☐ C treatment of acute infection is by passive immunisation
- ☐ D interferon gamma is a recognised treatment of the chronic carrier state
- ☐ E anti-HBs antibodies suggest a chronic carrier state has developed following acute infection

73. Concerning hepatitis A

- ☐ A chronic liver disease commonly follows acute infection
- ☐ B it is transmitted by the faeco-oral route
- ☐ C passive immunisation produces life-long immunity to infection
- ☐ D it is an RNA virus
- ☐ E diagnosis of acute infection is by stool culture

74. The following are likely to cause bloody diarrhoea:

- ☐ A rotavirus infection
- ☐ B *Campylobacter pylori* infection
- ☐ C ulcerative colitis
- ☐ D cystic fibrosis
- ☐ E *Giardia lamblia*

75. *Giardia lamblia*

☐ A is a bacteria
☐ B infestation is usually asymptomatic
☐ C can cause failure to thrive and chronic diarrhoea
☐ D symptomatic infection should be treated with erythromycin
☐ E can cause partial villous atrophy

76. Concerning intussusception

☐ A it is a known complication of Henoch-Schoenlein purpura
☐ B it is commonest in children under the age of 6 months
☐ C barium enema is contraindicated
☐ D if it presents over the age of 2 years an underlying cause is likely
☐ E pallor is often seen

77. Gilbert's syndrome

☐ A causes unconjugated hyperbilirubinaemia
☐ B causes bilirubinuria
☐ C can progress to cirrhosis
☐ D has a prevalence of 6%
☐ E episodes of jaundice are precipitated by acute infections

78. Features of ulcerative colitis include

☐ A arthropathy
☐ B transmural bowel inflammation
☐ C erythema nodosum
☐ D family history of inflammatory bowel disease
☐ E backwash ileitis

79. The following make a non-organic cause of recurrent abdominal pain more likely:

☐ A 3 year history
☐ B night pain
☐ C family history of migraine
☐ D mouth ulceration
☐ E weight loss

80. Pre-hepatic causes of portal hypertension include

☐ A Budd-Chiari syndrome
☐ B constrictive pericarditis
☐ C schistosomiasis
☐ D portal vein thrombosis
☐ E biliary atresia

81. Features of classical homocystinuria include

- ☐ A autosomal dominant inheritance
- ☐ B hyperextendable joints
- ☐ C normal at birth
- ☐ D predisposition to vascular thrombosis
- ☐ E aortic root dilatation

82. Congenital hypothyroidism

- ☐ A is usually due to dyshormonogenesis
- ☐ B is usually symptomatic in the neonatal period
- ☐ C incidence is 1 in 4000
- ☐ D high TSH, normal T4 on treatment suggests poor compliance
- ☐ E screening is at the 6 week check

83. Concerning Klinefelter's syndrome

- ☐ A karyotype is 47, XYY
- ☐ B increased risk of leukaemia
- ☐ C infertility is rare
- ☐ D gynaecomastia is a common finding in adolescents
- ☐ E testes are large

84. In Turner's syndrome

- ☐ A fetal loss in the first trimester is common
- ☐ B hypogonadotrophic hypogonadism is a feature
- ☐ C infants are usually born small for dates
- ☐ D spontaneous puberty is never seen
- ☐ E horseshoe kidney is a recognised association

85. Concerning phenylketonuria

- ☐ A the infant is normal at birth
- ☐ B the urine is odourless
- ☐ C it is caused by a deficiency of phenylalanine hydroxylase
- ☐ D seizures can occur
- ☐ E untreated individuals have a low IQ

86. Causes of a delayed bone age are

- ☐ A obesity
- ☐ B growth hormone deficiency
- ☐ C central precocious puberty
- ☐ D social deprivation
- ☐ E chronic asthma

87. Features of Noonan's syndrome include

- ☐ A webbing of the neck
- ☐ B pulmonary valve stenosis
- ☐ C mental retardation in 80%
- ☐ D delayed puberty
- ☐ E normal final adult height

88. Causes of gynaecomastia include

- ☐ A normal child
- ☐ B Klinefelter's syndrome
- ☐ C Noonan's syndrome
- ☐ D growth hormone deficiency
- ☐ E cimetidine

89. Features of Prader-Willi syndrome include

- [ ] A autosomal dominant inheritance
- [ ] B hypogonadism
- [ ] C hyperphagia
- [ ] D normal IQ
- [ ] E normal life expectancy

90. Concerning 21 hydroxylase deficiency

- [ ] A the gene defect is known
- [ ] B hypertension is common
- [ ] C a raised serum 17OH progesterone is characteristic
- [ ] D plasma chloride is low in salt losers
- [ ] E can present as precocious puberty in males

91. Growth hormone will increase the final adult height in the following circumstances:

- [ ] A growth hormone deficiency
- [ ] B familial short stature
- [ ] C hypothyroidism
- [ ] D Turner's syndrome
- [ ] E achondroplasia

92. The following are known to stimulate growth hormone secretion:

- [ ] A glucagon
- [ ] B arginine
- [ ] C aldosterone
- [ ] D thyroxine
- [ ] E insulin

93. Concerning central (true) precocious puberty

- [ ] A it is more common in boys than in girls
- [ ] B CT head scanning is indicated in all boys
- [ ] C it is usually idiopathic in girls
- [ ] D testicular volume would be expected to be increased in boys
- [ ] E it is gonadotrophin independent

94. Fragile X syndrome

- [ ] A occurs as a consequence of allelic expansion
- [ ] B is a cause of macro-orchidism in boys
- [ ] C is asymptomatic in carrier females
- [ ] D causes increasingly severe mental retardation with successive generations
- [ ] E is associated with small ears

95. Galactosaemia

- [ ] A has an incidence of 1 in 1000 live births
- [ ] B can cause congenital cataracts
- [ ] C can present with hypoglycaemia in the neonatal period
- [ ] D is associated with mental retardation even with early diagnosis
- [ ] E is treated with a lactose free diet

96. Aldosterone

- [ ] A secretion is stimulated by a fall in serum sodium
- [ ] B is secreted in response to a rise in blood pressure
- [ ] C deficiency is a cause of hypokalaemia
- [ ] D acts on the ascending limb of the loop of Henlé
- [ ] E levels are normal in pseudohypoaldosteronism

97. During puberty

- ☐ A   breast hypertrophy occurs in up to 40% of boys
- ☐ B   onset of the growth spurt in boys occurs at stage 4–5 of testicular enlargement
- ☐ C   peak height velocity in girls often occurs after menarche
- ☐ D   elongation of the eye can occur causing short sightedness
- ☐ E   the first sign of puberty in girls is the appearance of pubic hair

98. Insulin dependent diabetes (type one)

- ☐ A   has a peak incidence at 9–10 years of age
- ☐ B   is more common in children who possess the HLA-B3 antigen
- ☐ C   is associated with islet cell antibodies in 30% at diagnosis
- ☐ D   has a peak incidence during the summer months in the UK
- ☐ E   is associated with an increased risk of diabetes in siblings of the affected case

99. Complications of insulin dependent diabetes include

- ☐ A   tall stature
- ☐ B   hypoglycaemia
- ☐ C   lipoatrophy
- ☐ D   proximal myopathy
- ☐ E   cataract

100. Features of Graves' disease include

- ☐ A   inappropriate weight gain
- ☐ B   association with HLA DR3
- ☐ C   diarrhoea
- ☐ D   poor concentration
- ☐ E   male predominance

101. The following are used in the emergency treatment of hyperkalaemia:

☐ A   normal saline infusion
☐ B   intravenous salbutamol
☐ C   nebulised salbutamol
☐ D   intravenous adenosine
☐ E   intravenous hydrocortisone

102. Nocturnal enuresis

☐ A   the prevalence in 5 year olds is around 20%
☐ B   in children under the age of 10 is more common in boys than in girls
☐ C   the prevalence in 10 year olds is around 5%
☐ D   is primary in 95%
☐ E   the incidence is 10 times greater when either parent has had nocturnal enuresis

103. Berger's disease (mesangial IgA nephritis) is characterised by

☐ A   male predominance
☐ B   deafness
☐ C   exacerbations associated with upper respiratory infections
☐ D   end stage renal failure in 2 years
☐ E   proteinuria in 50%

104. In a 2-year-old pre-renal rather then renal failure is suggested by

☐ A   fractional excretion of sodium of 4%
☐ B   urinary sodium 10 mmol/l
☐ C   urine osmolality 250 mmol/l
☐ D   urine : plasma creatinine ratio of 5
☐ E   history of diarrhoea

105. Renal osteodystrophy

☐ A is a complication of chronic renal failure
☐ B is characterised by an increased plasma phosphate
☐ C is characterised by a reduced serum alkaline phosphatase
☐ D is characterised by a normal parathyroid hormone level
☐ E is familial

106. Renal involvement in Henoch-Schoenlein purpura

☐ A occurs in 25–50%
☐ B is always present within 4 weeks of the onset of the disease
☐ C usually manifests as an acute nephritis
☐ D is usually associated with a low C3 and C4
☐ E is usually progressive

107. The following patterns of inheritance are correct:

☐ A nephrogenic diabetes insipidus – autosomal recessive
☐ B Alport's syndrome – X linked dominant
☐ C Hartnup disease – X linked recessive
☐ D vitamin D resistant rickets (hypophosphataemic rickets) – autosomal dominant
☐ E cystinosis – X linked dominant

108. Minimal change nephrotic syndrome

☐ A has a peak incidence in children under 2 years
☐ B is commonly associated with macroscopic haematuria
☐ C has a male predominance
☐ D is usually associated with low C3
☐ E does not occur in adults

109. Metabolic acidosis occurs in

- ☐ A   pyloric stenosis
- ☐ B   cystinuria
- ☐ C   Bartter's syndrome
- ☐ D   cystinosis
- ☐ E   pseudohypoaldosteronism

110. In urinary tract infection in children

- ☐ A   investigation is always required
- ☐ B   *E. coli* is the causative agent in 80%
- ☐ C   DTPA is the appropriate investigation to look for renal scars
- ☐ D   amoxycillin is a useful prophylactic agent
- ☐ E   nitrofurantoin is a useful prophylactic agent

111. In children with haemolytic uraemic syndrome

- ☐ A   the C3 is usually low
- ☐ B   mortality is less than 1%
- ☐ C   thrombocytopenia is common
- ☐ D   the blood film is usually diagnostic
- ☐ E   dialysis is required in 50%

112. The following features are characteristic of proximal renal tubular acidosis:

- ☐ A   metabolic acidosis
- ☐ B   inability to acidify the urine after an acid load
- ☐ C   the condition usually occurs in isolation
- ☐ D   high urinary pH
- ☐ E   failure of tubular reabsorption of bicarbonate

113. Orthostatic proteinuria

- [ ] A is benign
- [ ] B is only present when the patient is upright
- [ ] C can be large
- [ ] D is commonly familial
- [ ] E can be precipitated by upper respiratory tract infection

114. In the assessment of haematuria

- [ ] A hypercalciuria is a recognised cause
- [ ] B a family history of deafness suggests IgA nephropathy
- [ ] C coexistent proteinuria makes a renal parenchymal problem more likely
- [ ] D renal tract ultrasound is essential
- [ ] E measurement of C3 is not usually helpful

115. Causes of hypertension in infancy include

- [ ] A a small blood pressure cuff
- [ ] B coarctation of the aorta
- [ ] C 17OH progesterone deficiency
- [ ] D prazosin
- [ ] E hypovolaemia

116. Concerning post-streptococcal glomerulonephritis

- [ ] A it is characterised by a low C3 in the acute phase
- [ ] B it follows non-haemolytic streptococcal infection in 50% of cases
- [ ] C hypertensive encephalopathy is a recognised complication
- [ ] D treatment with penicillin reduces the time course of the illness
- [ ] E it usually occurs in children under the age of 2 years

117. Concerning undescended testis

- ☐ A more common in premature infants
- ☐ B by 12 months 5% remain outside the scrotum
- ☐ C orchidopexy can be safely left until the second decade
- ☐ D there is an increased risk of infertility
- ☐ E there is an increased risk of malignant change

118. The following are associated with an increased risk of Wilms' tumour:

- ☐ A cystinosis
- ☐ B aniridia
- ☐ C neurofibromatosis
- ☐ D tuberous sclerosis
- ☐ E Beckwith Wiedemann syndrome

119. Chloride

- ☐ A is a cation
- ☐ B serum levels are high in pyloric stenosis
- ☐ C serum levels are high in renal tubular acidosis
- ☐ D serum levels may rise if normal saline is infused
- ☐ E is lost in the stool in chloridorrhoea

120. Recognised causes of hyponatraemia include

- ☐ A diabetes insipidus
- ☐ B high solute diet
- ☐ C inappropriate antidiuretic hormone secretion
- ☐ D diuretics
- ☐ E cystic fibrosis

121. Membranous glomerulonephritis

- ☐ A accounts for 20–40% of adult nephrotic syndrome
- ☐ B can be associated with hepatitis A infection
- ☐ C is more common in males than in females
- ☐ D is not improved by steroids
- ☐ E can be secondary to systemic lupus erythematosus

122. Concerning polycystic kidney disease

- ☐ A it is X linked
- ☐ B it can present in the neonatal period
- ☐ C adult presentation is associated with progression to renal failure in many cases
- ☐ D ultrasound is not a useful investigation
- ☐ E liver involvement with cysts is common

123. Concerning vesico-ureteric reflux

- ☐ A it occurs in less than 5% of children who present with a confirmed urinary tract infection
- ☐ B it is a risk factor for urinary tract infection
- ☐ C it is an indication for prophylactic antibiotics in all cases
- ☐ D spontaneous remission is common
- ☐ E it can be diagnosed using a DMSA scan

124. The following cause hypercalciuria:

- ☐ A frusemide
- ☐ B William's syndrome
- ☐ C hypoparathyroidism
- ☐ D distal renal tubular acidosis
- ☐ E vitamin D deficiency

125. Features of Finnish type congenital nephrotic syndrome include

☐ A raised alphafetoprotein antenatally
☐ B usually presents between 6 and 12 months
☐ C good prognosis
☐ D steroids are useful
☐ E autosomal recessive inheritance

126. Iron deficiency anaemia

- ☐ A is characterised by a low serum iron and a low total iron binding capacity
- ☐ B is associated with pica
- ☐ C is prevented by the early introduction of cows' milk
- ☐ D never requires treatment under the age of 6 months
- ☐ E in childhood is associated with chronic blood loss in most cases

127. Concerning idiopathic thrombocytopenia in childhood

- ☐ A bed rest is indicated
- ☐ B bone marrow examination is essential
- ☐ C incidence is 1 in 1000 children per year
- ☐ D platelet transfusion is necessary if the platelet count falls below 20
- ☐ E intravenous immunoglobulin may be beneficial

128. Glanzmann's thrombasthenia

- ☐ A is inherited as an autosomal dominant
- ☐ B gene locus is known
- ☐ C platelet count is normal
- ☐ D requires long term steroid treatment
- ☐ E splenectomy may be beneficial

129. Features of hereditary spherocytosis include

- ☐ A splenomegaly
- ☐ B conjugated hyperbilirubinaemia
- ☐ C gallstones
- ☐ D haemolytic crises following fava bean ingestion
- ☐ E X linked inheritance

130. Features of Wiskott Aldrich syndrome include

- [ ] A   autosomal recessive inheritance
- [ ] B   normal platelet count
- [ ] C   T cell defect
- [ ] D   death from acute haemorrhage in 20%
- [ ] E   eczema

131. Concerning vitamin B12

- [ ] A   deficiency can cause ataxia
- [ ] B   pernicious anaemia commonly occurs following terminal ileal resection
- [ ] C   in deficiency the mean corpuscular volume is usually normal
- [ ] D   deficiency usually occurs in untreated coeliac disease
- [ ] E   extrinsic factor promotes absorption

132. Sickle cell disease

- [ ] A   is associated with an increased risk of gallstones
- [ ] B   is associated with an increased risk of nocturnal enuresis
- [ ] C   can be diagnosed antenatally
- [ ] D   is an indication for prophylactic penicillin
- [ ] E   is associated with episodes of acute anaemia

133. Concerning rhesus haemolytic disease

- [ ] A   it cannot occur in first born children
- [ ] B   it occurs as a consequence of the transplacental passage of IgM
- [ ] C   the most common antibody type is anti-D
- [ ] D   it can present as hydrops fetalis
- [ ] E   it is an indication for premature delivery

134. In the anaemia of chronic disease

☐ A the haemoglobin is usually less than 8 g/dl
☐ B the total iron binding capacity is raised
☐ C the anaemia is usually normocytic
☐ D the serum iron is usually reduced
☐ E iron supplements are contraindicated

135. Neonatal thrombocytopenia

☐ A is an indication for cerebral ultrasound
☐ B is an absolute indication for platelet transfusion after delivery
☐ C may be caused by toxoplamosis infection during pregnancy
☐ D can occur in infants born to mothers with SLE
☐ E may be associated with absent radii

136. Concerning blood transfusion

☐ A pyrexia is an absolute indication for stopping the transfusion
☐ B back pain is an indication of severe transfusion reaction
☐ C hyperkalaemia is a well recognised complication
☐ D white cell filters are indicated if the patient is having regular transfusions
☐ E hydrocortisone and antihistamines minimise mild transfusion reactions in patients having regular transfusions

137. Causes of neutropenia include

☐ A hyperglycinaemia
☐ B cytotoxic drug therapy
☐ C chronic granulomatous disease
☐ D Kostmann's syndrome
☐ E X linked hypogammaglobulinaemia

138. Causes of bone pain and anaemia include

- ☐ A vitamin C deficiency
- ☐ B neuroblastoma
- ☐ C Langerhans cell histiocytosis
- ☐ D acute lymphoblastic leukaemia
- ☐ E sickle cell disease

139. Features of acute lymphoblastic leukaemia in childhood include

- ☐ A an incidence of 1 in 3500 in the first 10 years of life
- ☐ B fever at presentation
- ☐ C neutropenia
- ☐ D a better prognosis if the age is less than 2 years at presentation
- ☐ E long term survival in 50%

140. Thrombocytosis (platelet count >400 x10^9/l) is seen in

- ☐ A the first week of Kawasaki's disease
- ☐ B iron deficiency anaemia
- ☐ C post-splenectomy patients
- ☐ D Bernard-Soulier syndrome
- ☐ E juvenile chronic arthritis

141. Aplastic anaemia can occur secondary to

- ☐ A radiation
- ☐ B chloramphenicol
- ☐ C hepatitis A
- ☐ D Epstein Barr virus
- ☐ E parvovirus infection

142. Diseases with an increased risk of malignancy include

- ☐ A ataxia telangiectasia
- ☐ B Bloom syndrome
- ☐ C xeroderma pigmentosum
- ☐ D Down's syndrome
- ☐ E Fanconi's anaemia

143. Features of von Willebrand's disease include

- ☐ A prolonged bleeding time
- ☐ B autosomal recessive inheritance
- ☐ C menorrhagia
- ☐ D normal platelet count
- ☐ E normal platelet aggregation with ristocetin

144. Causes of a prolonged bleeding time include

- ☐ A Bernard Soulier syndrome
- ☐ B Henoch-Schoenlein syndrome
- ☐ C haemophilia
- ☐ D von Willebrand's disease
- ☐ E idiopathic thrombocytopenic purpura

145. Concerning X linked agammoglobulinaemia

- ☐ A the gene locus is known
- ☐ B the thymus is hypoplastic or absent
- ☐ C T cell function is normal
- ☐ D IgA, G and M are all reduced
- ☐ E intravenous immunoglobulin therapy is indicated

146. Di George syndrome

- ☐ A   inheritance is autosomal recessive
- ☐ B   the thymus is hypoplastic or absent
- ☐ C   cardiac defects are common
- ☐ D   the lymphocyte count is always reduced
- ☐ E   hypocalcaemia is common

147. Osteosarcoma

- ☐ A   usually presents in the first decade
- ☐ B   outcome <10% survival overall
- ☐ C   usually occurs in the metaphyseal region of growing bones
- ☐ D   lung metastasis at presentation occur in 80%
- ☐ E   fever at presentation is common

148. In accidental iron ingestion

- ☐ A   hypotension may occur within 2 hours of ingestion.
- ☐ B   toxicity is unlikely if vomiting stops within 2 hours of ingestion
- ☐ C   abdominal X-ray is a useful investigation
- ☐ D   pyloric stenosis may present 2 weeks after ingestion
- ☐ E   lactic acidosis may occur 12 hours post-ingestion

149. Carbon monoxide

- ☐ A   combines with haemoglobin to form carboxyhaemoglobin
- ☐ B   shifts the oxygen dissociation curve to the left
- ☐ C   toxicity occurs if the carboxyhaemoglobin level is 3–5%
- ☐ D   toxicity causes headache
- ☐ E   increases the oxygen carrying capacity of the blood

150. In overdosage with tricyclic antidepressants

- ☐ A tachycardia usually precedes coma
- ☐ B dialysis is effective at removing the drug
- ☐ C death is usually due to cardiac arrhythmias
- ☐ D the pupils are dilated
- ☐ E multiple doses of charcoal therapy should not be used

151. Toxoplasmosis

- ☐ A usually presents with pyrexia and a rash
- ☐ B can cause chorioretinitis
- ☐ C has an 80% risk of infecting the fetus if the mother is infected during pregnancy
- ☐ D is a cause of atypical lymphocytosis
- ☐ E infection is best diagnosed by serology

152. Concerning *Streptococcus pneumoniae*

- ☐ A it is a Gram-positive organism
- ☐ B it is the commonest cause of meningitis in childhood
- ☐ C vaccination with Pneumovax is recommended in children with sickle cell disease
- ☐ D there are four different serotypes
- ☐ E it is the cause of Lyme disease

153. In atypical mycobacterial infection

- ☐ A contact tracing is essential
- ☐ B pulmonary involvement is more common in children than in adults
- ☐ C lymphoma is part of the differential diagnosis
- ☐ D incision and drainage is the recommended treatment of an infected node
- ☐ E anti-tuberculous chemotherapy is indicated in all cases

154. Familial Mediterranean fever

- ☐ A is inherited as an autosomal dominant
- ☐ B amyloidosis is a recognised complication
- ☐ C colchicine can be used to suppress an attack
- ☐ D is a bacterial infection
- ☐ E is characterised by episodes of abdominal pain and fever

155. Which of the following are DNA containing viruses:

☐ A   mumps
☐ B   hepatitis B
☐ C   molluscum contagiosum
☐ D   hepatitis C
☐ E   respiratory syncitial virus

156. Which of the following statements regarding CSF are correct:

☐ A   a normal CSF glucose excludes bacterial meningitis
☐ B   red cells are a normal finding in the CSF of a child over the age of 6 years
☐ C   CSF protein is higher in the neonate than in the older child
☐ D   a spinal cord tumour can cause a lymphocytosis
☐ E   the white cell count is always raised in bacterial meningitis

157. Impetigo

☐ A   is contagious
☐ B   is best treated with topical antibiotics
☐ C   can cause a bullous rash
☐ D   causes a fever in the majority of cases
☐ E   is usually due to staphylococcal infection

158. Features of infectious mononucleosis include

☐ A   spread is by transmission of oral secretions
☐ B   heterophile antibodies in the blood
☐ C   positive Paul Bunnell in all cases
☐ D   atypical lymphocytosis
☐ E   splenomegaly

159. Concerning schistosomiasis

- ☐ A it is usually asymptomatic
- ☐ B it is a cause of obstructive uropathy
- ☐ C chronic granulomatous injury occurs with chronic infection
- ☐ D terminal haematuria is typical of *Schistosoma haematobium*
- ☐ E mebendazole is the drug of choice

160. The following are notifiable diseases:

- ☐ A respiratory syncitial virus positive bronchiolitis
- ☐ B mumps
- ☐ C yellow fever
- ☐ D hepatitis A
- ☐ E meningococcal septicaemia

161. Concerning measles

- ☐ A it is a DNA virus
- ☐ B Koplik's spots are pathognomonic
- ☐ C it is most contagious during the prodromal period
- ☐ D a fatal carditis can occur
- ☐ E a single vaccination provides lifelong immunity

162. Concerning Lyme disease

- ☐ A transmission to humans is by infected ticks
- ☐ B erythema toxicum is characteristic
- ☐ C it can present with a 7th nerve palsy
- ☐ D antibiotics are unhelpful
- ☐ E diagnosis is usually made on blood culture

163. Concerning parvovirus B19 infection

- ☐ A it is a cause of non-immune hydrops
- ☐ B it can cause aplastic crises in sickle cell disease
- ☐ C thrombocytopenia is a recognised complication
- ☐ D intravenous immunoglobulin is indicated in all cases
- ☐ E an arthropathy can occur

164. Concerning the vertical transmission of hepatitis B

- ☐ A it is more likely if the mother is hepatitis B 'e' antigen positive
- ☐ B it is reduced by passive immunisation at birth
- ☐ C active immunisation is affected by maternal IgG
- ☐ D active and passive immunisation is more protective than passive immunisation alone
- ☐ E vertical transmission occurs around the time of birth

165. Factors that suggest transient synovitis of the hip joint rather than septic arthritis include

- ☐ A age less than 5 years
- ☐ B normal ESR
- ☐ C normal hip radiograph
- ☐ D neutrophilia
- ☐ E pyrexia

166. Risk factors for the vertical transmission of HIV include

- ☐ A advanced clinical disease in the mother
- ☐ B high CD4 count
- ☐ C preterm delivery
- ☐ D Caesarian section
- ☐ E prolonged rupture of membranes

167. The following are causes of erythema nodosum:

☐ A tuberculosis
☐ B systemic lupus erythematosus
☐ C inflammatory bowel disease
☐ D Hodgkin's disease
☐ E streptococcal infection

168. Concerning systemic lupus erythematosus

☐ A antibodies to double stranded DNA are virtually diagnostic
☐ B 50% are ANA negative
☐ C a low C3 suggests renal disease
☐ D Ro/SSA is suggestive of neonatal lupus
☐ E procainamide can induce ANA positivity

169. Concerning Perthes' disease

☐ A it predominantly occurs in males
☐ B it is always unilateral
☐ C patients are usually older than 10 years at presentation
☐ D the incidence is 1 in 2000
☐ E obesity is common

170. The following are true regarding immunisations:

☐ A MMR vaccine should not be given to HIV positive children
☐ B live polio vaccine should not be given to siblings of children receiving chemotherapy
☐ C pertussis vaccine is contraindicated if there is a first degree relative with convulsions
☐ D MMR vaccine is ineffective if given within 3 months of immunoglobulin therapy
☐ E influenza vaccination is not indicated in children with cystic fibrosis

171. The following are recognised side effects of the following vaccinations:

☐ A   collapse following the acellular pertussis vaccine
☐ B   parotid swelling in the third week after MMR
☐ C   convulsions following pertussis
☐ D   poliomyelitis following the Salk poliovirus vaccine
☐ E   regional adenitis following BCG

172. Concerning influenza immunisation

☐ A   anaphylactic hypersensitivity to egg protein is a contraindication
☐ B   routine immunisation of health care workers is recommended
☐ C   the vaccine is live
☐ D   the vaccine is given by intradermal injection
☐ E   cystic fibrosis is a contraindication

173. Diseases associated with HLA B27 include

☐ A   ankylosing spondylitis
☐ B   diabetes mellitus
☐ C   psoriatic arthropathy
☐ D   Marfan's syndrome
☐ E   dermatomyositis

174. Characteristic early features of Kawasaki's disease include

☐ A   exudative conjunctivitis
☐ B   thrombocytosis
☐ C   palmar erythema
☐ D   lymphadenopathy
☐ E   coronary artery thrombosis

175. Complications of rubella infection include

☐   A   orchitis
☐   B   thrombocytopenic purpura
☐   C   arthritis
☐   D   encephalitis
☐   E   congenital cataract

176. The following are useful in the assessment of gestational age in preterm infants:

☐ A   presence of palmar creases
☐ B   breast size
☐ C   sacral oedema
☐ D   the scarf sign
☐ E   muscle tone

177. The following statements about pulmonary hypertension are true:

☐ A   it is a recognised complication of group B streptococcal sepsis
☐ B   hyperventilation is an effective treatment
☐ C   tolazoline is a potent pulmonary vasoconstrictor
☐ D   radial arterial PaO_2 is lower then umbilical artery PaO_2
☐ E   birth asphyxia is a risk factor

178. Concerning air leak syndromes in the newborn

☐ A   an underwater seal drain is only required if the pneumothorax is under tension
☐ B   in a term baby with a small pneumothorax giving oxygen at high concentration can worsen it
☐ C   increasing the I:E ratio in a ventilated baby decreases the risk of pneumothorax
☐ D   pneumomediastinum is usually fatal
☐ E   they can be asymptomatic

179. Recognised problems of infants born at term small for gestational age include

☐ A   hypothermia
☐ B   sepsis
☐ C   polycythaemia
☐ D   hypoglycaemia
☐ E   retinopathy of prematurity

180. Complications of steroid therapy in the newborn include

- ☐ A leucopenia
- ☐ B hypoglycaemia
- ☐ C cataracts
- ☐ D sepsis
- ☐ E gastric perforation

181. Concerning necrotising enterocolitis

- ☐ A exchange transfusion is a predisposing factor
- ☐ B *Clostridium welchii* is implicated in the pathogenesis
- ☐ C it is most common in infants born less than 1500 g
- ☐ D oral antibiotics are useful
- ☐ E complications include short bowel syndrome

182. The following statements are true:

- ☐ A fracture of the cervical spine can occur with breech deliveries
- ☐ B waiter's tip positioning of the arm is seen with Klumpke's paralysis
- ☐ C phrenic nerve palsy with diaphragmatic weakness occurs with Erb's palsy
- ☐ D caput succedaneum is limited by suture lines
- ☐ E the clavicle is the commonest bone to fracture during labour and delivery

183. Causes of recurrent apnoeas in preterms include

- ☐ A sepsis
- ☐ B gastro-oesophageal reflux
- ☐ C bowel movement
- ☐ D hypoglycaemia
- ☐ E anaemia

184. Concerning respiratory distress syndrome

☐ A   maternal diabetes is a risk factor
☐ B   it is characterised by reduced lung compliance
☐ C   it is treated with surfactant given down the endotracheal tube
☐ D   prognosis is better in males
☐ E   steroids given within 4 hours of delivery reduce the incidence of respiratory distress syndrome

185. Phototherapy

☐ A   reduces serum unconjugated bilirubin levels
☐ B   is a substitute for exchange transfusion in small preterms
☐ C   is not very effective in dark skinned infants
☐ D   can cause watery stools in the treated infant
☐ E   increases fluid requirements

186. Infants of diabetic mothers

☐ A   usually develop hypoglycaemia on the second day of life
☐ B   are always large for gestational age
☐ C   sacral agenesis is one of the congenital anomalies seen
☐ D   are at increased risk of developing diabetes mellitus
☐ E   have an increased incidence of respiratory distress syndrome

187. Concerning neonatal polycythaemia

☐ A   it refers to a haemoglobin level of above 180 g/l
☐ B   trisomy 21 is a predisposing factor
☐ C   necrotising enterocolitis is a recognised complication
☐ D   capillary packed cell volume is usually less than venous packed cell volume
☐ E   there are no long term complications

188. The following statements are true about perinatal asphyxia:

- ☐ A   multiple gestation is a risk factor
- ☐ B   it is the commonest cause of cerebral palsy in the UK
- ☐ C   persistent fetal circulation is a recognised complication
- ☐ D   seizures occur in grade I hypoxic ischaemic encephalopathy
- ☐ E   hypocalcaemia can occur

189. Bile stained vomit on the first day of life

- ☐ A   makes duodenal atresia unlikely
- ☐ B   with a history of meconium-stained amniotic fluid rules out intestinal obstruction
- ☐ C   suggests pyloric stenosis
- ☐ D   requires a barium enema to rule out malrotation
- ☐ E   if due to meconium ileus responds to gastrograffin enemas in half the cases

190. The following statements are true:

- ☐ A   cord haemoglobin in a term infant is usually between 12 and 14 g/dl
- ☐ B   increased red cell breakdown is the main cause of the physiological anaemia of infancy
- ☐ C   fetal haemoglobin does not have a beta chain
- ☐ D   beta thalassaemia can present with anaemia in the neonatal period
- ☐ E   the Apt test differentiates fetal from maternal haemoglobin

191. Problems associated with preterm gestation include

- ☐ A   pulmonary haemorrhage
- ☐ B   hyperglycaemia
- ☐ C   jaundice
- ☐ D   metabolic acidosis
- ☐ E   periventricular leucomalacia

192. Causes of neonatal fits include

- ☐ A   Wilson's disease
- ☐ B   hypoglycaemia
- ☐ C   Di George syndrome
- ☐ D   lead poisoning
- ☐ E   kernicterus

193. Risk factors for congenital dislocation of the hip include

- ☐ A   breech delivery
- ☐ B   spina bifida
- ☐ C   male sex
- ☐ D   positive family history
- ☐ E   being first born

194. Predominantly conjugated hyperbilirubinaemia occurs with the following:

- ☐ A   breast milk jaundice
- ☐ B   Crigler-Najjar syndrome
- ☐ C   biliary atresia
- ☐ D   alpha-1 antitrypsin deficiency
- ☐ E   choledochal cyst

195. Chickenpox in the neonate

- ☐ A   is a contraindication to breast feeding
- ☐ B   requires treatment with i.v. aciclovir
- ☐ C   is infectious
- ☐ D   has a mortality untreated of 90%
- ☐ E   is suggestive of an underlying immunodeficiency

COMMUNITY PAEDIATRICS AND CHiLD PSYCHIATRY

196. Concerning anorexia nervosa

- ☐ A it is more common in pupils of fee-paying schools
- ☐ B concordance is higher in monozygotic twins than in dizygotic twins
- ☐ C it is rarely associated with depression
- ☐ D continuing weight loss is an indication for hospital admission
- ☐ E less than 1% of cases are boys

197. Concerning childhood autism

- ☐ A there is an increased incidence of epilepsy in adolescence
- ☐ B it is caused by poor parenting
- ☐ C Asperger's syndrome represents a sub-group with more severe disease
- ☐ D it is more common in girls
- ☐ E 20% of cases are associated with a medical disorder

198. Concerning hyperkinetic disorder of childhood

- ☐ A it is successfully controlled by dietary restriction
- ☐ B it can lead to poor academic achievement
- ☐ C it can be exacerbated by anticonvulsant treatment
- ☐ D it is commoner in boys
- ☐ E the use of drug therapy commonly causes sleep disturbance

199. School refusal

- ☐ A is different from truancy
- ☐ B is commonly associated with physical symptoms
- ☐ C is associated with anxiety and depression
- ☐ D can be treated with antidepressants
- ☐ E generally has a poor outcome

200. Concerning childhood squints

☐ A they occur in 4% of pre school-children
☐ B they often causes amblyopia of the affected eye
☐ C they are an absolute indication for tests of visual acuity
☐ D paralytic squint is more common than non-paralytic squint
☐ E non-paralytic squints rarely require corrective surgery

201. In the assessment of hearing

☐ A a history of cleft palate is relevant
☐ B pure tone audiometry testing can be used in children of any age
☐ C auditory brain stem evoked responses are affected by sedation
☐ D deafness may be associated with a family history of sudden death
☐ E a history of prematurity is significant

202. Munchausen's by proxy

☐ A should be suspected in cases of childhood hypoglycaemia
☐ B has about a 10% risk to the child of death or disability
☐ C is more common in pre-verbal children
☐ D is associated with a family history of sudden infant death
☐ E symptoms do not occur when the parent or primary care giver is away from the child

203. Psychiatric referral is indicated for

☐ A a 15-year-old girl who has taken an overdose of paracetamol
☐ B a 14-year-old boy off school with recurrent morning headaches
☐ C grief reaction in a 6-year-old boy lasting for a year
☐ D a 9-year-old who is afraid of the dark
☐ E encopresis in a 7-year-old boy where constipation has been excluded

204. In childhood depression

- [ ] A   sleep is characteristically increased
- [ ] B   a family history is common
- [ ] C   girls are more likely to have depression than boys at all ages
- [ ] D   auditory hallucinations are a recognised feature
- [ ] E   parasuicidal behaviour is very rare

205. Concerning sudden infant death syndrome

- [ ] A   prematurity is a risk factor
- [ ] B   the risk is increased with increasing maternal age
- [ ] C   it is more common in females
- [ ] D   it is associated with paternal smoking
- [ ] E   it is associated with sleeping on plastic mattresses

206. Concerning child sexual abuse

- [ ] A   it occurs in up to 10% of children
- [ ] B   child sexual abusers often have a history of being abused as a child
- [ ] C   girls are 20 times more likely to be abused than boys
- [ ] D   it is associated with an increased incidence of anal fissures
- [ ] E   reflex anal dilatation is pathognomonic

207. Concerning physical abuse in children

- [ ] A   fathers are more likely to be abusers than mothers
- [ ] B   it is more common in first born children
- [ ] C   handicapped children are at increased risk
- [ ] D   the head and neck are the commonest sites of injury
- [ ] E   the majority of non-accidental fractures occur in children of school age

208. Concerning childhood schizophrenia

- ☐ A it is rare
- ☐ B long term remission occurs in 90%
- ☐ C delusions are a feature
- ☐ D family history is often positive
- ☐ E it is associated with a lifetime increased risk of suicide

209. Speech delay is

- ☐ A more common in females
- ☐ B common in autism
- ☐ C associated with tongue tie
- ☐ D more common in first born children
- ☐ E associated with a family history of speech delay

210. Causes of developmental regression include

- ☐ A Down's syndrome
- ☐ B cerebral palsy
- ☐ C Gaucher's disease
- ☐ D subacute sclerosing panencephalitis
- ☐ E HIV infection

211. A child of 8 months would be expected to

- ☐ A transfer from hand to hand
- ☐ B roll from back to front
- ☐ C build a tower of 3 bricks
- ☐ D say two words with meaning
- ☐ E sit without support

212. A child of 18 months would be expected to

☐ A throw a ball without falling
☐ B spontaneously scribble
☐ C wave bye bye
☐ D feed with a spoon
☐ E speak in sentences

213. A child of 3 years would be expected to

☐ A copy a square
☐ B name two colours
☐ C ride a tricycle
☐ D go up stairs one foot per step
☐ E build a tower of six cubes

214. A child of 12 months would be expected to

☐ A pick up a sugar cube between the finger and thumb
☐ B be dry during the day
☐ C feed with a biscuit
☐ D use at least two different words with meaning
☐ E wave bye bye

215. Causes of toe walking include

☐ A habit
☐ B peroneal muscular atrophy
☐ C spastic diplegia
☐ D spina bifida
☐ E tendo-achilles shortening

216. Concerning Guillain-Barre syndrome

- [ ] A implicated infectious agents include Coxsackie virus
- [ ] B distal sensory loss may occur
- [ ] C reduced reflexes are present
- [ ] D weakness is usually asymmetrical
- [ ] E autonomic involvement does not occur

217. In spinal muscular atrophy type I (Werdnig-Hoffmann disease)

- [ ] A inheritance is usually autosomal recessive
- [ ] B the genetic abnormality is localised to chromosome 5
- [ ] C the usual presentation is with delayed walking
- [ ] D creatinine phosphokinase is always raised
- [ ] E survival beyond 3 months is rare

218. Concerning epilepsy

- [ ] A in a complex seizure consciousness is lost
- [ ] B simple refers to short duration
- [ ] C partial seizures begin focally
- [ ] D epilepsy that is difficult to control is classified as symptomatic
- [ ] E an aura is necessary to make a diagnosis

219. Features of tuberous sclerosis include

- [ ] A 50% recurrence risk in offspring
- [ ] B adenoma sebaceum
- [ ] C hypsarrhythmic change on the EEG
- [ ] D good response of seizures to treatment with vigabatrin
- [ ] E the frequent occurrence of malignant tumours

220. Concerning cerebral palsy

☐ A   75% of cases are idiopathic
☐ B   birth weight of less than 1500 g is a risk factor
☐ C   mental retardation occurs in 20%
☐ D   perinatal asphyxia accounts for more than 50%
☐ E   prevalence is 1%

221. Features of petit mal epilepsy (typical absence epilepsy of childhood) include

☐ A   age less than 2 years
☐ B   characteristic inter-ictal EEG
☐ C   good response to carbamazepine
☐ D   long term remission
☐ E   long term risk of generalised seizures

222. The following are causes of cerebral palsy:

☐ A   hypothyroidism
☐ B   preterm delivery
☐ C   Werdnig-Hoffmann disease
☐ D   neonatal meningitis
☐ E   congenital cytomegalovirus infection

223. Concerning infantile spasms

☐ A   they occur in the first year of life
☐ B   EEG findings are non-specific
☐ C   the symptomatic group has a worse prognosis
☐ D   vigabatrin is frequently used as the drug of first choice
☐ E   30% of cases are idiopathic

224. Causes of hypotonia in the infant include

☐ A Becker's muscular dystrophy
☐ B failure to thrive
☐ C subacute sclerosing panencephalitis
☐ D coeliac disease
☐ E Down's syndrome

225. Features of a parietal lobe lesion include

☐ A contralateral homonymous hemianopia
☐ B disinhibition
☐ C grasp reflex
☐ D receptive dysphasia
☐ E apraxia

226. Benign rolandic epilepsy

☐ A represents less than 1% of childhood epilepsy
☐ B carries a poor prognosis
☐ C abnormal inter-ictal EEG
☐ D nocturnal generalised seizures can occur
☐ E there is a good response of seizures to sodium valproate

227. Manifestations of a third nerve palsy include

☐ A ptosis
☐ B pupil dilatation
☐ C blindness
☐ D diplopia
☐ E failure of lateral gaze

228. Concerning Friedrich's ataxia

- ☐ A   the gene locus is known
- ☐ B   plantars are down going
- ☐ C   a third of patients develop malignancy
- ☐ D   onset is usually by the age of five
- ☐ E   pes cavus is a recognised finding

229. The following conditions are inherited as autosomal dominant:

- ☐ A   tuberous sclerosis
- ☐ B   ataxia telangiectasia
- ☐ C   colour blindness
- ☐ D   haemophilia
- ☐ E   myotonic dystrophy

230. In Duchenne muscular dystrophy

- ☐ A   inheritance is autosomal recessive
- ☐ B   creatinine phosphokinase is usually elevated
- ☐ C   muscle biopsy is unhelpful
- ☐ D   the defect is on chromosome 6
- ☐ E   cardiac involvement can occur

231. Risk factors for simple febrile convulsions include

- ☐ A   age less than 6 months
- ☐ B   family history of epilepsy
- ☐ C   family history of febrile convulsions
- ☐ D   past history of urinary tract infection
- ☐ E   previous febrile convulsion

232. Concerning complex partial seizures (temporal lobe epilepsy)

- ☐ A consciousness is impaired
- ☐ B ethosuximide is the drug of first choice
- ☐ C the EEG shows three per second spikes
- ☐ D they can present as drop attacks
- ☐ E they are the commonest form of childhood epilepsy

233. Myoclonic jerks are commonly seen in

- ☐ A Lennox-Gastaut syndrome
- ☐ B Janz syndrome
- ☐ C Landau-Kleffner syndrome
- ☐ D West's syndrome
- ☐ E Gilbert's syndrome

234. The radial nerve

- ☐ A supplies the small muscles of the hand
- ☐ B nerve root is T1
- ☐ C is responsible for elbow extension
- ☐ D lesion is called Klumpke's paralysis
- ☐ E palsy causes wrist drop

235. The following statements are true concerning primitive reflexes:

- ☐ A it is normal for the Moro reflex to be present at 8 months of age
- ☐ B the palmar grasp reflex usually disappears by three months of age
- ☐ C persistence of the asymmetric tonic neck reflex is an early sign of cerebral palsy
- ☐ D the parachute reflex is present at birth
- ☐ E the plantar reflex is normally flexor by 4 weeks

236. The following conditions are associated with hydrocephalus:

- ☐ A anaemia
- ☐ B Klippel-Feil syndrome
- ☐ C choroid plexus papilloma
- ☐ D Dandy Walker malformation
- ☐ E mucopolysaccharidoses

237. Which of the following conditions are associated with microcephaly:

- ☐ A malnutrition
- ☐ B holoprosencephaly
- ☐ C meningitis
- ☐ D trisomy 13
- ☐ E thyrotoxicosis

238. Regarding brain tumours

- ☐ A change in personality can be the presenting feature
- ☐ B craniopharyngiomas can present with a visual field defect
- ☐ C metastatic tumours are common in childhood
- ☐ D oligodendrogliomas are the commonest brain tumour in childhood
- ☐ E brain tumours are the commonest malignancy in childhood

239. Concerning neurofibromatosis

- ☐ A acoustic neuromas are present in type one
- ☐ B maternal folate deficiency is a risk factor
- ☐ C optic nerve gliomas are seen
- ☐ D it is usually associated with intellectual impairment
- ☐ E type 2 is commoner then type one

240. The following are causes of facial weakness:

- ☐ A hypertension
- ☐ B Epstein Barr virus
- ☐ C Erb's palsy
- ☐ D birth injury
- ☐ E myasthenia gravis

1. NEONATAL CYANOSIS   Answer: DE

The hyperoxia test is used to help differentiate between cardiac and non-cardiac causes of cyanosis. Cyanosis is indicative of more than 5 g/dl of haemoglobin being in the reduced state. The test is performed as follows: once cyanosis is confirmed by either an arterial blood gas or pulse oximetry the infant is given 100% oxygen to inspire. The baby with a respiratory cause for cyanosis will generally show a good increment (PaO_2 > 20 kPa) whereas the infant with cyanotic congenital heart disease and a right to left shunt will not. There are some exceptions to this including total anomalous pulmonary venous drainage (due to pulmonary oedema) in which a moderate but not complete response to the hyperoxia test will be seen.

Acrocyanosis is peripheral cyanosis of the hands, feet and occasionally trunk. It is very common in the first 24 hours of life.

If a duct-dependent cardiac lesion is suspected then a prostaglandin infusion should be started which prolongs patency of the ductus arteriosus pending transfer to a cardiac unit. Side effects of prostaglandin include apnoea and therefore the child needs to be ventilated.

Differential diagnosis of cyanosis in the newborn
Cardiac causes
Respiratory disease
CNS depression
Methaemoglobinaemia
Narcotics e.g. pethidine

Methaemoglobinaemia
The iron of both oxygenated and deoxygenated blood is normally in the ferrous state – this is essential for its oxygen transporting function. Oxidation of the haemoglobin iron to the ferric state yields methaemoglobin. Methaemoglobin is non-functional and can in sufficient quantities cause cyanosis. It imparts a brown colour to the blood. Methaemoglobinaemia can be hereditary or acquired. Acquired methaemoglobinaemia occurs secondary to ingestion of substances that oxidise haemoglobin including dapsone, chloroquine and nitrites. Treatment is with ascorbic acid and methylene blue.

2. DOWN'S SYNDROME

Answer: BD

Cardiac lesions in Down's syndrome

Cardiac lesions are present in 30–50% of children with Down's syndrome. Of these defects, 30% are atrioventricular septal defects (AVSD) and 30% are isolated ventricular septal defects. Other cardiac lesions commonly seen include tetralogy of Fallot and patent ductus arteriosus. 25% of all children with an AVSD have Down's syndrome. All children with Down's syndrome should have an echocardiogram.

Pulmonary vascular disease in children with Down's syndrome

There is an increased incidence of pulmonary vascular disease in children with Down's syndrome. The principal aetiology is cardiac (increased pulmonary flow). Other contributing factors include upper airway obstruction (laryngomalacia and adenotonsillar hypertrophy) and an increased incidence of intrinsic lung disease.

Atrioventricular septal defect

= endocardial cushion defect
Atrioventricular septal defects (AVSD) can be classified as partial or complete. In the partial form an ostium primum ASD is present with or without a cleft in the mitral valve. In the complete form there is a common atrio-ventricular valve with clefts in both the pulmonary and mitral valves.

3. TRANSPOSITION OF THE GREAT ARTERIES

Answer: ABDE

Transposition of the great arteries (TGA) represents about 6 % of all congenital heart disease. It is the commonest cause of cyanotic congenital heart disease in the neonatal period. It is more common in males than females.

In TGA the aorta arises from the right ventricle and carries deoxygenated blood to the body, the pulmonary artery arises from the left ventricle and carries oxygenated blood to the lung. A lesion that mixes the two circulations is essential for survival (examples include patent ductus arteriosus, atrioventricular septal defect, ventricular septal defect). The child is usually cyanotic from or shortly after birth. The lesion is duct dependent and the infant deteriorates when the duct closes. There is usually a metabolic acidosis at presentation. Arrhythmias of all types are common. ECG shows a right sided axis and right ventricular hypertrophy. The chest X-ray shows cardiomegaly and an increased pulmonary vascularity.

Surgical management of TGA
- Palliative – atrial septostomy
- Physiological repair (permanent palliation) – Mustard, Senning
- Anatomical – Jatene arterial switch (corrective)
            – Rastelli's (conduit – needs replacement)

4. TETRALOGY OF FALLOT   Answer: BE

This accounts for 10% of congenital heart disease.

Components of Tetralogy of Fallot
Ventricular septal defect
Right ventricular outflow obstruction
Right ventricular hypertrophy
Overriding aorta

The severity of the right ventricular outflow obstruction will determine the clinical picture.
- Mild obstruction – pink Fallot's – left to right shunt across the ventricular septal defect – murmur ejection systolic (pulmonary stenosis) – become cyanotic later as the shunt reverses
- Moderate obstruction – presents with cyanosis – right to left shunt across VSD – murmur is ejection systolic due to pulmonary stenosis, VSD silent
- Severe obstruction – duct dependent, presenting with cyanosis in the neonatal period

ECG shows right ventricular hypertrophy and right axis deviation in cyanotic Fallot's. The ECG in acyanotic Fallot's shows right ventricular hypertrophy because the right ventricular pressure is high.

Cyanotic spells usually begin around 4–6 months of age. They are
- due to functional infundibular spasm
- potentially fatal
Features include worsening cyanosis and a reduction in the intensity of the murmur.

Treatment of cyanotic spells
Bring baby's knees to chest (reduces venous return)
Beta blockers
Morphine
Sodium bicarbonate if acidotic
Vasoconstrictors

Surgical management of Fallot's is either palliative (systemic to pulmonary shunt) or complete. Total correction, if technically possible, is the preferred option. This is usually done at around 6 months.

Complications of Fallot's
Polycythaemia
Subacute bacterial endocarditis
Cerebral abscess, cerebral thrombosis
Retardation of growth and development
Clubbing – usually appears after 1 year of age.

5. NEONATAL CYANOSIS — Answer: BCDE

Eisenmenger's syndrome is an acquired defect secondary to pulmonary hypertension. Cyanosis occurs in the hypoplastic left heart syndrome secondary to circulatory failure and worsens when the duct closes. Severe (critical) aortic stenosis can present in the neonatal period with cyanosis by the same mechanism.

Cardiac conditions presenting with neonatal cyanosis
Decreased pulmonary flow
    Pulmonary atresia
    Fallot's tetralogy
    Ebstein's anomaly
Increased pulmonary flow
    Hypoplastic left heart
    Tricuspid atresia
    Truncus arteriosus
    Total anomalous pulmonary venous drainage
    Double outlet ventricle
    Single ventricle
Poor mixing
    Transposition of the great arteries

6. PAEDIATRIC ECGs — Answer: ABCE

Mean QRS
At birth   125 degrees
1 month   90 degrees
3 years   50 degrees
The right axis deviation seen in newborns is due to right ventricular dominance in the fetus.

Right bundle branch block

Right bundle branch block is the commonest conduction disturbance seen in children. The abnormality is usually due to right ventricular overload prolonging right ventricular depolarisation due to lengthening of the conduction pathway.

Criteria for right bundle branch block

Prolonged QRS
Right axis deviation
Terminal slurring of the QRS over the right ventricular leads V3R, V4R and V1
ST depression and T wave inversion is commonly seen in adults but rarely in children

Causes of right bundle branch block

Atrioventricular septal defect
Ebstein's anomaly
Coarctation of the aorta (infants)
Endocardial cushion defects
Post right ventriculotomy
Partial anomalous pulmonary venous drainage
Normal variant

Congenital heart block

Congenital complete heart block (i.e. complete atrioventricular dissociation) occurs in infants of mothers with systemic lupus erythematosus, particularly those with anti Ro (SS-A) and anti La (SS-B) antibodies. The damage to the conduction pathway is irreversible. Antenatal diagnosis is possible because of persistent fetal bradycardia. 50% have an associated structural defect, usually congenitally corrected transposition. The condition is usually well tolerated and often does not require a pacemaker.

QT prolongation

Romano Ward – autosomal dominant
Jervell Lange Nielsen syndrome – autosomal recessive (associated with congenital deafness)
These are important causes of sudden death in previously healthy young persons.

Heart rate

Heart rate varies with the age and status of the patient. A rate of 110–150 is normal in the newborn and the adult rate of 60–100 is achieved by the age of 6 years.

Wolff-Parkinson-White syndrome
Patients with this syndrome are prone to supraventricular tachycardia from pre-excitation due to an anomalous atrioventricular conduction pathway.

The ECG characteristics include:

*   Shortened PR interval
*   Prolonged QRS
*   Delta wave – slurring of the upstroke to the QRS complex.

There is a recognised association with Ebstein's anomaly.

7. CHEST X-RAYS   Answer: CDE

Coeur en sabot ('heart in a boot')
This is seen in tetralogy of Fallot and is due to hypoplasia of the main pulmonary artery and the consequent up turning of the apex away from the diaphragm. A right-sided aortic arch is seen in 25%.

Rib notching
This is a feature of coarctation of the aorta and occurs as a consequence of the increase in size of the intercostal vessels which function as collaterals. The upper two or three ribs are spared because their posterior intercostal arteries do not arise from the aorta. Rib notching is rarely seen in children under the age of 5 years.

Other chest X-ray changes of coarctation
*   Dilation of the ascending aorta, descending aorta (post stenotic dilatation)
*   Cardiomegaly
*   Increased pulmonary vascular shadowing

Truncus arteriosus
The features on chest X-ray include a right-sided aortic arch, absent thymus (30% of cases have Di George syndrome), cardiomegaly, and a prominent ascending aorta.

Total anomalous pulmonary venous drainage

There are two types of TAPVD:

- Unobstructed – cardiomegaly, increased pulmonary vascular markings
- Obstructed – normal heart size, increased pulmonary vascular markings (severe pulmonary oedema)

The lesion may be supra-cardiac, cardiac, infra-cardiac or mixed. Obstructed lesions are usually infra-cardiac. In the supra-cardiac unobstructed total anomalous pulmonary venous drainage, dilation of the left and right superior vena cavae and the left innominate vein give rise to a 'cottage loaf' or 'snowman' appearance on chest X-ray.

Scimitar syndrome

This is a form of partial anomalous pulmonary venous drainage whereby the veins from the right lung drain directly into the inferior vena cava. The right lung is hypoplastic as a consequence and this allows movement of the heart to the right. The single vein draining the right lung produces a scimitar shape on the PA chest X-ray as it heads towards the right cardio-diaphramatic angle.

8. **CONDITIONS ASSOCIATED WITH AN INCREASED RISK OF HEART DISEASE**   **Answer: ABCD**

Kawasaki's disease

The cardiac lesions appear in the second week of the illness as proximal coronary artery aneurysms healing by fibrosis and thrombosis. Lesions are most common on the left side. Protection is offered by the early administration of intravenous immunoglobulin. Other cardiac lesions can occur including aortic and mitral regurgitation, myocarditis, pericarditis, pericardial effusion and myocardial infarction.

Congenital rubella

Infection with rubella during the first trimester causes the classical triad of deafness, cataracts and cardiac anomalies. Cardiac defects include peripheral pulmonary artery stenosis, patent ductus arteriosus and septal defects. Other abnormalities seen in the congenital rubella syndrome include microcephaly, microphthalmia, intra-uterine growth retardation, hepatitis and neonatal thrombocytopenia.

Marfan's syndrome

Mitral valve prolapse
Dilation/dissection of the ascending aorta
Aortic regurgitation

Pulmonary artery aneurysm
Mitral valve regurgitation

Turner's syndrome

The commonest cardiac lesion is coarctation of the aorta (15–30%). Other cardiac lesions seen include aortic stenosis, atrioventricular septal defect, and bicuspid aortic valves. Hypertension is not uncommon. Lesions commonly seen in Noonan's syndrome include pulmonary stenosis and obstructive cardiomyopathy. For examination purposes it is worth remembering that in Noonan's syndrome right-sided heart lesions are seen and in Turner's syndrome left-sided heart lesions are seen.

There is no increase in the incidence of congenital heart disease in petit mal epilepsy.

9. CONGENITAL HEART DISEASE   Answer: CE

The commonest congenital heart disease is a ventricular septal defect.

The lung fields are oligaemic in tetralogy of Fallot.

Blalock-Taussig Shunt

This is an anastomosis between the subclavian artery and the pulmonary artery and is used for palliation of tetralogy of Fallot. The murmur is continuous. Continuous murmurs characteristically pass through the second heart sound into diastole.

Ebstein's Anomaly

This is displacement of the septal and posterior leaflets of the tricuspid valve causing atrialisation of part of the right ventricle. In severe cases, children can present with cyanosis and cardiac failure. Arrhythmias are common including Wolf-Parkinson-White. Lithium during pregnancy is a risk factor.

Nitric and not nitrous oxide is used to treat persistent pulmonary hypertension.

Causes of plethoric lung fields
Acyanotic
    Atrioventricular septal defect
    Ventricular septal defect
    Patent ductus arteriosus (PDA)

Endocardial cushion defect
Partial anomalous pulmonary venous drainage
Cyanotic
Single ventricle
Truncus arteriosus
Hypoplastic left heart
Transposition of the great arteries
Total anomalous pulmonary venous drainage

Causes of continuous murmurs
Blalock-Taussig shunt
AV malformation
Aneurysm
Collateral vessels
PDA
Venous hum
Peripheral pulmonary stenosis

10. ATRIAL SEPTAL DEFECTS   Answer: ABE

Isolated atrial septal defects (ASDs) account for 8% of congenital heart disease. The defect is commoner in females and there are three types:
* Ostium secundum (commonest)
* Ostium primum
* Sinus venosus

Ostium secundum defects are usually asymptomatic with pulmonary hypertension and right ventricular failure occurring in the third and fourth decades. Atrial arrhythmias occur in adulthood but are rare in childhood. Antibacterial prophylaxis is unnecessary for a secundum ASD. An ostium primum defect is likely to present earlier usually as a component of an endocardial cushion defect and does require antibiotic prophylaxis.

ECG appearance of atrial septal defects
Ostium primum – right bundle branch block, left axis deviation
Ostium secundum – right bundle branch block, right axis deviation
The presence of right bundle branch block is not diagnostic but its absence makes the diagnosis unlikely.

A high proportion of ostium secundum ASDs close spontaneously by the age of 5 years. The risk of pulmonary hypertension and its sequelae increases with shunt size. Surgical repair is indicated if the pulmonary to systemic flow ratio is greater than 2:1. High pulmonary vascular resistance is a contraindication to surgery.

Fixed splitting of the second heart sound is characteristic of an ASD. This is due to the defect producing a constantly increased right ventricular volume and prolonging ejection time.

The murmur of an ASD is not due to flow across the defect but due to increased flow across the pulmonary valve as a consequence of the shunt.

11. VENTRICULAR SEPTAL DEFECTS   Answer: D

Ventricular septal defects are the commonest congenital heart defect. The defect can occur in the membranous or muscular part of the septum. Defects in the membranous septum are more common and are usually single. Defects in the muscular part of the septum are usually multiple.

The signs and symptoms depend on the haemodynamics of the defect, which is dependent on the size of the defect and the pulmonary vascular resistance. With a small defect, the murmur is rarely present at birth but appears as the pulmonary vascular resistance falls.

Untreated, a large shunt will result in high pulmonary flow and can progress to pulmonary hypertension and the Eisemenger's syndrome. The second heart sound is loud if pulmonary hypertension is present.

Infective endocarditis occurs in less than 2% of cases.

It is the left and not the right ventricle that is volume overloaded. The shunt occurs mainly during systole when the right ventricle is contracting, and so the shunted blood enters the pulmonary circulation.

The right atrium contains deoxygenated blood, the right ventricle contains deoxygenated blood from the right atrium and oxygenated blood from the left ventricle. At cardiac catheterisation, the oxygen content of blood in the right ventricle is greater than that in the right atrium.

30–60% close spontaneously in the first 6 months and many more subsequent to that. Surgery is required if the left to right shunt is such (usually quoted as > 2:1) that pulmonary hypertension has or is likely to develop.

12. EISENMENGER'S SYNDROME   Answer: BDE

Eisenmenger's syndrome is pulmonary hypertension at a systemic level due to fixed elevation of pulmonary vascular resistance (i.e. pulmonary vascular disease) with a reversed or bi-directional shunt at the atrial, ventricular or aorto-pulmonary level.

Cardiac defects associated with the development of Eisenmenger's syndrome include any cause of increased pulmonary artery flow with increased pulmonary artery pressure:
- Ventricular septal defect (VSD)
- Atrioventricular septal defect (ASD)
- Patent ductus arteriosus (PDA)
- Aortopulmonary window
- Total anomalous pulmonary venous drainage
- Truncus arteriosus
- Endocardial cushion defects
- Double outlet right ventricle
- Transposition of the great arteries with a VSD

Symptoms of pulmonary vascular disease do not usually develop until the second or third decade. The following are risk factors for the earlier development of pulmonary hypertension:
- Cardiac defect with large shunt
- Perinatal asphyxia
- Recurrent chest infections
- Chronic upper airway obstruction
- Down's syndrome
- Birth at or living at high altitude

Symptoms and signs of Eisenmenger's syndrome
- Dyspnoea
- Syncope
- Haemoptysis
- Arrhythmias
- Clubbing
- Raised jugular venous pressure
- Right ventricular heave
- Loud P2

Heart–lung transplant is the only surgical option.

Cardiac abnormalities presenting with cyanosis and reduced pulmonary flow are protected from the development of pulmonary vascular disease – pulmonary atresia, pulmonary stenosis, tetralogy of Fallot.

Pulmonary valve stenosis is associated with
Noonan's syndrome
Trisomy 18
Fetal valproate syndrome
Maternal rubella
Neurofibromatosis
Leopard syndrome
William's syndrome

Critical/severe pulmonary stenosis presents in the neonatal period with cyanosis and right-sided heart failure which worsens with duct closure. Arrhythmias are common. Management is difficult and has high morbidity and mortality. The treatment of choice is stabilisation with prostaglandin followed by balloon dilatation or surgery.

13. PATENT DUCTUS ARTERIOSUS   Answer: ABE

This accounts for 5–10% of congenital heart defects excluding extremely preterm infants. It is present in 40–50% of preterm infants whose birth weight is less than 1750 g, 30% of which have a significant ductus with congestive cardiac failure. The reason for the higher incidence in preterm infants is that the responsiveness of ductal smooth muscle is gestation dependent.

In term infants functional closure occurs within 10–15 hours of birth with complete anatomical closure by 2–3 weeks of age.

Presentation of PDA in the preterm infant
Cardiac failure
Apnoea
Increased ventilatory requirements

Presentation of PDA in the term infant
Small shunt
   asymptomatic
Large shunt
   poor weight gain
   tachypnoea

tachycardia
cardiac murmur

Findings on examination
Continuous machinery murmur
Full pulses
Loud P2
In the preterm infant the murmur may be limited to systole.

Management of PDA
In the preterm infant this is dependent upon symptoms. Spontaneous closure is likely if the duct is asymptomatic. In symptomatic infants the management is fluid restriction, diuretics, maintenance of normal haemoglobin, indomethacin and surgical ligation.
In the term infant indomethacin is not helpful and the principal therapeutic option is surgical with a catheter closure of the duct being performed between 6 months and 2 years of age. Spontaneous closure is not likely in term infants (persistence of the duct for 3 months = persistent ductus arteriosus).

14. FETAL CIRCULATION   Answer: None correct

Oxygenated blood from the placenta returns to the fetus via the umbilical vein. 50% enters the hepatic circulation and 50% bypasses the liver via the ductus venosus.

Most of the inferior caval blood as it enters the right atrium is directed through the foramen ovale into the left atrium. The right atrium contains blood from the superior vena cava, coronary sinus and some from the inferior vena cava. Right atrial blood enters the right ventricle. 85% of right ventricular blood passes into the descending aorta via the ductus arteriosus, 15% enters the fetal lungs.

Changes in the fetal circulation occur at birth. The ductus venosus closes and loss of the low resistance placenta results in an increase in systemic vascular resistance. There is a functional closure of the foramen ovale. Lung expansion results in a fall in pulmonary vascular resistance, increased pulmonary blood flow and increased delivery of blood to the left atrium. Flow through the ductus arteriosus changes from the pulmonary to systemic to the systemic to pulmonary circulation. The high concentration of oxygen in the blood causes smooth muscle contraction of the duct and closure.

15. CONGENITAL HEART DISEASE
Answer: CE

Poor growth (height and weight) is common in children with cyanotic congenital heart disease. Catch-up growth after corrective surgery is common.

The contraindications to immunisation are as for the normal population.

The oral contraceptive pill is contraindicated in girls with cyanotic congenital heart disease due to the risk of thrombosis. The coil is also contraindicated as it is a potential focus of infection predisposing to endocarditis.

6–10% of children with congenital heart disease have a chromosomal abnormality. 30% of newborn infants with chromosomal abnormalities have heart defects.

16. COARCTATION OF THE AORTA
Answer: ACE

This accounts for 10% of congenital heart disease. It is commoner in males (2:1). Associated cardiac anomalies include
- Bicuspid aortic valve (70%)
- Mitral valve disease
- Sub aortic stenosis
- Ventricular septal defect

The coarctation is usually just after the origin of the left subclavian artery (98%) at the level of the ductus arteriosus. It can occur proximal to the origin of the left subclavian artery in which case the blood pressure in the right arm will be higher than in the left arm; the classical discrepancy being between the upper and lower limb blood pressure. The murmur of coarctation is systolic. Continuous murmurs are occasionally heard from collaterals. Up to 10% of children with coarctation have berry aneurysms in the cerebral circulation.

Rib notching does not appear until late childhood.

Treatment is surgical by either balloon dilatation, graft or a subclavian flap. This is usually carried out soon after diagnosis.

Associations of coarctation of the aorta
Trisomy 13
Trisomy 18
Turner's syndrome
Valproate toxicity

Aortic valve stenosis
This accounts for 5% of congenital heart defects. It is commoner in males. Associations include:
- William's syndrome
- Turner's syndrome
- fetal phenytoin syndrome.

The stenosis can be either supravalvular, valvular or subvalvular. There is often an associated bicuspid valve.

Aortic stenosis is usually asymptomatic but in its most severe form can cause congestive cardiac failure, arrhythmias and sudden death in infancy (rare).

The murmur is best heard in the aortic area and radiates to the neck. An ejection click suggests valvular stenosis. A palpable thrill is usually present in the suprasternal notch.

Although left ventricular hypertrophy is common the ECG can be normal.

Surgery includes valvotomy, balloon dilatation and valve replacement and is indicated if the peak systolic pressure between the left ventricle and aorta is greater then 60 mmHg.

Assessment of severity
1 Symptoms – angina like pain
                      – syncopy/dizziness on exertion
                      – palpitations on exertion
2 ECG evidence of left ventricular strain
3 Exercise test positive
                      – ST and T wave changes on the ECG during exercise

17. TERATOGENS   Answer: ABDE

The following are teratogens for the defects shown

Alcohol	ASD, VSD, PDA, TGA
Amphetamines	ASD, VSD, PDA, TGA
Lithium	Ebstein's anomaly
Oestrogens/progesterones	VSD, TGA, Fallot's
Phenytoin	Pulmonary stenosis, aortic stenosis, PDA, Coarctation, ASD, VSD
Thalidomide	Fallot's, truncus arteriosus
Sodium valproate	Aortic stenosis
Warfarin	Fallot's, VSD

18. HYPERTENSION   Answer: None correct

Childhood hypertension is defined as systolic or diastolic blood pressure greater then the 95th centile for age, recorded on three separate occasions.

There are two types, primary (aetiology unknown) and secondary (aetiology known). Secondary hypertension is commoner in infants and younger children. Primary hypertension is more common than secondary hypertension in adolescents and young adults when there is often a family history.

Children with primary hypertension are rarely symptomatic. Obesity is associated with primary hypertension.

70–80% of children with secondary hypertension have a renal cause. Initial investigations are aimed at detecting renal parenchymal disease.

19. CIRCULATORY FAILURE IN THE FIRST   Answer: ABCDE
WEEK OF LIFE

Cardiac Causes
Critical aortic stenosis
Hypoplastic left heart
Coarctation
Myocardial ischaemia (hypoxic ischaemic encephalopathy, hypoglycaemia)
Severe anaemia

Cardiomyopathy
Arrhythmia
Arteriovenous fistula
Obstructed pulmonary venous drainage
Transposition of the great arteries with VSD

By the end of the first week when pulmonary vascular resistance falls left to right shunts become an important cause of heart failure including ventricular septal defect, patent ductus arteriosus, atrioventricular septal defect and truncus arteriosus. Non-cardiac causes of heart failure such as sepsis and fluid overload need to be considered.

20. INFECTIVE ENDOCARDITIS   Answer: None correct

The most common organism is *Streptococcus viridans*. Other causes include *Staphylococcus aureus* and *Enterococcus*. The infected lesions are usually left sided (apart from those in intravenous drug abusers).

Most patients who develop infective endocarditis have either congenital or acquired heart defects. With the exception of an ostium secundum atrioventricular septal defect all congenital heart defects increase the risk of endocarditis. The commonest source of the bacteria is the teeth. Good dental hygiene and antibiotic prophylaxis for dental procedures is essential.

The clinical manifestations are often difficult and non-specific. More than 80% have a fever. 50% have skin manifestations which include petechiae, Osler's nodes and splinter haemorrhages. 50% have embolic phenomena. Haematuria is common. Finger clubbing may occur in chronic cases. A murmur is universal – either a new murmur or the change in character of an existing murmur.

Diagnosis is on clinical suspicion, positive blood culture (which may need to be done repeatedly – three blood cultures 95% pick up rate) and by the demonstration of valvular vegetations on echocardiography.

Treatment is with long-term antibiotics. Surgery is occasionally required.

21. CARDIOMYOPATHY   Answer: AB

Hypertrophic
60% of cases of hypertrophic cardiomyopathy are inherited as an

autosomal dominant. Of these, 50% are due to mutations of the beta cardiac myosin heavy chain genes. These patients can be detected using polymerase chain reaction prior to the onset of symptoms. Infants of diabetic mothers and infants on steroids for chronic lung disease experience a transient form. Sudden death occurs in 4–6% of affected children per year.

Dilated
Idiopathic/multifactorial is the commonest form. There is an X linked type that presents in adolescence. The commonest cause is idiopathic (probably post viral). Other causes include adriamycin toxicity, phaeo-chromocytoma, mitochondrial disease and carnitine deficiency.

Restrictive
This is very rare in childhood. Associations include sarcoidosis, amyloidosis, haemochromatosis, Fabry's disease and Loeffler's syndrome.

Endocardial fibroelastosis
This is a form of dilated cardiomyopathy. Usually only the left side of the heart is affected. There are both hereditary and non-hereditary forms. This is very rare in childhood.

Infants of diabetic mothers have a three times greater risk of congenital heart disease than the rest of the population. Defects seen include ventricular septal defect, transposition, coarctation, persistent pulmonary hypertension, reversible hypertrophic cardiomyopathy.

22. RHEUMATIC FEVER   Answer: AB

Rheumatic fever develops secondary to infection with group A beta-haemolytic *Streptococcus*. It is commoner in lower socio-economic classes and the peak incidence is between the ages of 5 and 15.

Rheumatic fever is diagnosed by the Duckett Jones criteria:
Major criteria

Carditis	50%
Chorea	15%
Polyarthritis	70%
Erythema marginatum	10%
Subcutaneous nodules	1%

Minor criteria
   Arthralgia
   Fever
   Prolonged PR interval
   Raised ESR, CRP

Diagnosis is dependent on two major or one major and two minor criteria being present and there being evidence of recent streptococcal infection (raised ASO titres, antideoxyribonuclease B). The exceptions are

- Chorea – if no other cause is identifiable then chorea by itself is diagnostic
- Insidious/late onset carditis with no other explanation
- Rheumatic recurrence – the presence of one major or one minor criterion with evidence of prior streptococcal infection suggests recurrence.

Pancarditis occurs in 50%. Consequences of this include heart block, tachycardia, cardiomegaly, congestive cardiac failure and valve disease. It is only the carditis that produces sequelae which include mitral regurgitation, mitral stenosis, aortic regurgitation and tricuspid regurgitation.

Aspirin is indicated in the acute phase, initially at 120 mg/kg for 14 days and then 70 mg/kg until the fever settles. Prednisolone is indicated in severe carditis. Antibiotic prophylaxis should be continued long term.

23. INNOCENT MURMURS

Answer: CE

Features of an innocent murmur
Localised
Poorly conducting
Musical/vibratory
Soft grade 1–3/6 *
Systolic *
Varies with posture
Present in high output states e.g. febrile illness
Cardiac examination otherwise normal
Chest X-ray, ECG normal
*except venous hum

Still's murmur

This is an early systolic murmur most commonly heard in children aged 2–6 years resolving towards adolescence. Grade 1–3 present in early systole, heart sounds normal. Maximum intensity is at lower left sternal edge. The murmur is vibratory and best heard with the patient flat reducing in intensity when they sit up.

Venous hum

This is a continuous murmur most commonly heard in children aged 2–6 years. The diastolic component is usually loudest. It is best heard over the supraclavicular fossa on the right with the head turned to the other side. It may radiate and is often heard on both sides. It disappears on lying flat or if the neck veins are compressed.

Pulmonary flow murmur

This is a very common murmur. Characteristically it is brief and in mid systole. It is loudest with the patient supine and during expiration. Occurs in children and adolescents of all ages and is louder during hyperdynamic states such as fever and post exercise.

Innocent murmurs are commonly heard in the neonatal period.

24   CARDIAC EMERGENCIES   Answer: E

Supraventricular tachycardia

The commonest cardiac arrythmia in the paediatric age group is a supraventricular tachycardia. Classically the onset is abrupt. It can last for a few minutes or several days. It is tolerated well by most children although the majority will develop cardiac failure if the arrhythmia persists for long enough.

Management depends on whether the child is in shock as a consequence of the arrhythmia. Options include:
- Vagal stimulation – facial immersion/carotid massage
- Adenosine (can cause apnoea) – bolus doses given into a proximal vein – 50 µg/kg, 100 µg/kg, 250 µg/kg.
- Digoxin, flecainide
- Synchronous DC shock

Management of asystole/electromechanical dissociation

Clear airway
Ventilation with high concentration oxygen and cardiac massage

Adrenaline – i.v. endotracheal, intraosseus
Fluid expansion
Further adrenaline
Exclude tamponade, pneumothorax, drug overdose

Asystole is the commonest arrest rhythm in childhood.

Ventricular fibrillation
This is rare in childhood. Potential causes include tricyclic antidepressant toxicity, hypothermia, hyperkalaemia, myocarditis and myocardial infarction. Treatment is by asynchronous DC shock (after a praecordial thump) at 2 J/kg. This is repeated at the same dose if no output is produced and the dose then doubled. Adrenaline is given if there is still no response. A resuscitation circuit is then established including CPR, DC shock and adrenaline which is continued either until a response is obtained or resuscitation discontinued. All resuscitation drugs can be given intraosseusly except bretylium tosylate which is an anti-arrhythmic occasionally used in older children.

25. ECG   Answer: ADE

The PR interval varies with age.
*   Upper limit of normal in infants   0.14 s
*   Upper limit of normal in older children   0.16 s

The QT interval varies with heart rate.
*   Upper limit of normal under 6 months   0.49 s
*   Upper limit of normal over 6 months   0.44 s

Myxomas are the commonest adult cardiac tumour. They are rare in childhood. They are most commonly found in the left atrium. Rhabdomyomas are the commonest cardiac tumours in childhood. These are usually located on the ventricular septum and may be multiple. They are associated with tuberous sclerosis. They can cause obstruction to ventricular flow and arrythmias. Spontaneous regression does occur.

Cerebral abscess is rare under the age of 2 years. Cerebral thrombi are more common (albeit still very rare).

The third heart sound occurs as a consequence of rapid ventricular filling during diastole. It occurs in up to 20% of normal children. It is loud in conditions with decreased ventricular compliance secondary to ventricular dilatation, for example cardiac failure secondary to a ventricular septal defect.

Causes of a prolonged PR interval
Atrioventricular septal defect
AV canal defect
Ebstein's anomaly
Myocarditis
Ischaemia
Hypothermia
Hyperkalaemia
Duchenne muscular dystrophy
Digoxin
Quinidine

Causes of a prolonged QT interval
Hypocalcaemia
Hypothyroidism
Hypothermia
Myocarditis
Severe malnutrition
Romano Ward syndrome
Jervell Lange Nielson syndrome
Head injury
Cerebrovascular accident
Drugs – erythromycin, quinidine, procainamide

26. LYMPHOCYTIC INTERSTITIAL PNEUMONITIS   Answer: AE

Lymphocytic interstitial pneumonitis is defined as reticulonodular pulmonary infiltrates that persist for 2 months or more, with or without associated lymphadenopathy, that do not respond to antimicrobials in an HIV-infected patient. It is an AIDS defining diagnosis.

It occurs in 15% of children with vertically acquired HIV infection. The aetiology is not known but coexistent infection with Epstein-Barr virus may have a role. The onset is usually insidious but can be acute and rarely presents before the age of two. The disease can be asymptomatic. Early symptoms are of dry cough and exertional dyspnoea. Long standing disease is accompanied by finger clubbing and chronic bronchiectasis. Acute deterioration of chronic disease occurs with super-imposed bacterial or viral infections. In this instance, hypoxia and respiratory decompensation can occur.

The chest X-ray appearance is of hilar lymphadenopathy with diffuse bilateral interstitial infiltrates more prominent in the lower lobes. Other causes of interstitial infiltrates include tuberculosis, cytomegalovirus infection and *Pneumocystis* infection. A lung biopsy is occasionally required for the diagnosis.

Treatment with AZT is not of proven benefit. For severe disease, treatment should be with high dose oral steroids for 6–12 weeks followed by a maintenance dose with oxygen therapy if required.

27. THEOPHYLLINE   Answer: CD

Increased clearance	Decreased clearance
Cigarette smoking	Prematurity
Phenytoin	Obesity
Phenobarbitone	Cirrhosis
Alcohol	Congestive cardiac failure
Rifampicin	Fever
Carbamazepine	Acute viral illness
	Pneumonia
	Cimetidine
	Erythromycin
	Ciprofloxacin
	Allopurinol
	Verapamil
	Propranolol

28. *PNEUMOCYSTIS CARINII* PNEUMONIA   Answer: DE

Pneumocystis carinii has attributes of fungi and protozoa. *Pneumocystis carinii* pneumonia occurs in 40% of children with AIDS. It is most common in the first year of life when it is associated with a poor outcome. Overall the mortality from childhood infection is high. Signs and symptoms are often non-specific and diagnosis is often delayed. The chest X-ray may be normal or show a diffuse interstitial infiltrate. Diagnosis is by isolation of the organism from respiratory secretions or lung biopsy. Treatment is with co-trimoxazole and steroids. Prophylaxis is given to HIV-infected infants routinely.

Extrapulmonary infection is rare (retina, spleen, bone marrow).

80% of children with HIV infection develop pulmonary disease. The most important respiratory pathologies are *Pneumocystis carinii* pneumonia, lymphocytic interstitial pneumonitis and tuberculosis. The incidence of normal childhood respiratory illness is also increased. The CD4 count is a good marker of immune dysfunction and the risk of opportunistic infection rises as it falls. *Mycobacterium tuberculosis* infection is common in HIV-infected children. The tuberculin skin test is often negative but the response to therapy good.

29. ASTHMA   Answer: ABCD

Pulsus paradoxus is the difference between systolic blood pressure in inspiration and expiration. Patients with a difference greater than 20 mmHg have severe asthma or cardiac tamponade.

Pulse oximetry is a good indicator of the severity of an acute attack of asthma. It is also a good predictor of the duration of the attack if done on admission to hospital with an episode of acute asthma.

Features of severe asthma
Inability to talk in sentences
Intercostal recession
Peak flow less than 50% expected
Reduced level of consciousness
Oxygen saturation less than 85% in air
Silent chest
Cyanosis

30. PULMONARY HYPOPLASIA   Answer: ABDE

Pulmonary hypoplasia occurs in 1 in 1000 births. It can be unilateral or bilateral. Causes can be primary (rare) or secondary.

Reduced volume of the affected hemithorax
Congenital diaphragmatic hernia
Pleural effusion
Thoracic dystrophy
Congenital cyst

Oligohydramnios
Prolonged rupture of membranes
Potter's syndrome
Renal tract anomalies

Reduced pulmonary vascular perfusion
Hypoplastic left heart
Pulmonary artery agenesis
Tracheo-oesophageal fistula

Outcome is variable. Babies who are ventilated have a high risk of pulmonary interstitial emphysema.

Unilateral hypoplasia usually presents late and can be asymptomatic.

Potter's syndrome
This is a sporadic condition and consists of oligohydramnios with consequent pulmonary hypoplasia. In its most severe form the oligohydramnios is due to renal agenesis. The baby has a classic appearance with a squashed face, hypertelorism, prominent epicanthic folds, micrognathia, low set ears and large floppy hands and feet. All of these babies die although some survive for up to 48 hours.

Other developmental anomalies of the lung
Congenital lung cysts
Cystic adenomatoid malformation
Congenital lobar emphysema
Lobar sequestration

31. ACUTE STRIDOR IN CHILDHOOD   Answer: ABE

Causes
Acute laryngotracheobronchitis
Acute epiglottitis
Foreign body
Bacterial tracheitis
Retropharyngeal abscess
Tonsillitis (quinsy)
Angioneurotic oedema
Diphtheria
Thermal, mechanical (e.g. post extubation) or chemical trauma

Steroids and croup
Recent evidence suggests that it is beneficial to give nebulised steroid (as budesonide) on admission to children with croup (acute laryngotracheo-bronchitis) and that this both shortens the illness and reduces disease severity. In severe croup intravenous steroids
• reduce the need for intubation
• reduce the duration of intubation and ventilation if required
• reduce the incidence of subglottic stenosis in ventilated babies.

Adrenaline and croup
Nebulised adrenaline 1 ml of 1 in 1000 solution will provide temporary relief in croup lasting 20–30 minutes. Other therapies, such as steam, although widely used are not of proven benefit.

32. BRONCHIOLITIS   Answer: ADE

50–70% of cases are due to respiratory syncitial virus infection. Other aetiological agents include adenovirus, parainfluenza virus, rhinovirus, mumps, influenza virus and *Mycoplasma pneumoniae.*

It is most common during the first 6 months of life. Peak incidence in the winter months. Risk factors include maternal smoking, poor social circumstances, not being breast fed and male sex.

Inappropriate antidiuretic hormone secretion can occur during the acute phase of the illness.

Treatment is mainly supportive. Nebulised ipratropium bromide or nebulised salbutamol may be beneficial. Antibiotics are only indicated for secondary bacterial infection. Steroids are unhelpful. Ribovarin is probably of benefit in selected cases including children with pre-existing cardiac or respiratory disease such as bronchopulmonary dysplasia or congenital heart disease. There is no vaccine of proven efficacy. Passive immunisation with hyperimmune immunoglobulin has been carried out in the United States.

The neutrophil count is usually normal. Chest X-ray shows hyper-inflation with scattered areas of atelectasis in 30%. Respiratory syncitial virus can be demonstrated in nasopharyngeal secretions.

Complications during the acute phase include
- difficulty feeding
- apnoea
- bacterial infection
- respiratory failure.

Recurrent wheeze post-bronchiolitis occurs in 40–50%. Duration of attack, family history of asthma and cigarette smoking are risk factors.

33. RESPIRATORY FAILURE   Answer: BDE

Type I
Reflects ventilation perfusion mismatch and presents with hypoxia and normo- or hypocapnia.
Aetiologies include:
- Pulmonary oedema
- Pneumonia
- Pulmonary embolus
- Acute asthma
- Adult respiratory distress syndrome

Type II
Reflects hypoventilation and presents with hypoxia and hypercapnia.
Aetiologies include:
- Head injury/encephalitis/meningitis
- Muscle disease
- Drugs
- Kyphoscoliosis
- Severe asthma
- Respiratory obstruction
- Pneumothorax

Patients with type I respiratory failure can progress to type II when respiratory muscle fatigue occurs or with CNS depression from hypoxia.

34. LARYNGOMALACIA (CONGENITAL LARYNGEAL STRIDOR)

Answer: A

In infancy 60–70% of persistent stridor is due to laryngomalacia. This usually presents at birth, but can present at any stage up to 4 weeks. Most children with laryngomalacia thrive and feed normally. The condition usually resolves by 18 months of age.

Specific indications for investigation include stridor at rest, late presentation (>4 months) and failure to thrive. In addition any stridor that is persistent, severe and biphasic should be further investigated. Investigations that should be considered include chest X-ray, lateral neck X-ray, barium swallow and direct laryngoscopy.

The aetiology is unknown, with histologically normal cartilage.

Differential diagnosis of laryngomalacia
Neonatal tetany
Subglottic stenosis
Subglottic haemangioma
Laryngeal nerve palsy
Laryngeal web
Vascular ring
Congenital floppy larynx
Goitre

35. ASTHMA

Answer: ABDE

Salmeterol is a long-acting beta stimulant. It is useful for prominent night cough, exercise-induced symptoms and as an add on treatment in refractory chronic asthma when control is poor despite other therapies. The duration of action following administration is 12 hours.

Fluticasone propionate is a corticosteroid which exhibits almost complete first-pass metabolism in the liver and therefore has minimal systemic absorption. It is available in inhaler and dischaler form.

Sodium cromoglycate inhaled shortly before exercise can prevent exercise-induced asthma.

36. BRONCHOSCOPY   Answer: AE

Bronchoscopy can be carried out with either a flexible or a rigid endoscope. A rigid endoscope is an open tube and therefore a child can be ventilated through it. It can be left *in situ* and is therefore appropriate for the removal of foreign bodies, clots and mucous plugs and in massive haemoptysis. A flexible endoscope is solid and requires ventilation to occur around it. There is a suction and biopsy channel – larger objects cannot be removed through it. Bronchoscopy can be either diagnostic or therapeutic.

Indications for bronchoscopy
Diagnostic
    Congenital stridor
    Foreign body
    Persistent atelectasis
    Unexplained interstitial disease
    Undiagnosed infection particularly in an immunocompromised host
    Haemoptysis
Therapeutic
    Bronchopulmonary lavage
    Removal of clot, mucous plug, foreign body

Investigation of suspected foreign body
Clinical history of inhalation.
Inspiratory/expiratory films or screening to look for unilateral hyper-inflation.
Ventilation perfusion scan
Bronchoscopy
Fluoroscopy

Commonest site of impaction is the right main stem bronchus.

Complications of bronchoscopy
Hypoxia
Cardiac arrhythmias
Bronchospasm
Laryngospasm
Infection
Haemorrhage
Pneumothorax

37. SWEAT TEST   Answer: BC

The sweat test is the most appropriate diagnostic test for cystic fibrosis. Diagnostic values are of a sweat sodium greater than 70 mmol/l or a sweat chloride of greater than 70 mmol/l on a sample weighing more than 100 mg. A number of books quote a sweat chloride of greater than 60 mmol/l as being diagnostic. Three tests should be performed to confirm the diagnosis. In normal individuals the sodium is greater than the chloride and the sum of the two is less than 140 mmol/l. In patients with cystic fibrosis the chloride is usually greater than the sodium and the sum greater than 140 mmol/l. In the general population over the age of 16, 10% have a sweat sodium greater than 60 mmol/l. In these patients a fludrocortisone test can be performed in order to confirm the diagnosis.

Plasma immunoreactive trypsin (IRT) is useful until the age of 3 months. Pancreatic function tests are sometimes required and typically show normal enzyme values with a low bicarbonate concentration.

A number of children with cystic fibrosis get a pseudo-Bartter's syndrome with hyponatraemia and hypokalaemia due to excessive salt losses in the sweat.

Causes of a raised sweat sodium
Cystic fibrosis
Adrenal insufficiency
Pseudohypoaldosteronism
Hypothyroidism
Nephrogenic diabetes insipidus
Glycogen storage disease type one
Mucopolysaccharides
Glucose 6 phosphate dehydrogenase deficiency
Nephrotic syndrome
Severe malnutrition
HIV infection

Causes of a false-negative sweat test
Oedema
Hypoproteinaemia

38. CLEFT LIP AND PALATE   Answer: ADE

This is a defect of mesodermal development. The lips usually fuse between the 5th and 7th weeks of gestation and the palate between the 9th and 12th. Antenatal ultrasound is helpful. Cleft lip can be detected by skilled operators by 17 weeks. Cleft palate is more difficult to see.

The incidence is 1 in 700 births. Cleft lip 1 in 600, cleft palate 1 in 1000. The recurrence risk if there is an affected sibling is 1 in 25. If one parent is affected the risk is 1 in 20.

Cleft lip and palate is an isolated abnormality in 75%. A third of patients have cleft lip only and a quarter have cleft palate only. Associations are more common in children with cleft palate alone (20–50%) than children with cleft lip only (7–13%) or cleft lip and palate (2–11%). Submucous cleft palate (3% of all clefts) is suggested by a bifid uvula and central translucent zone in the palate.

Problems associated with cleft lip and palate
Feeding difficulties with poor weight gain
Difficulty with bonding
Respiratory disease
Speech delay
Hypernasal speech
Glue ear with impaired hearing
Dental caries
Problems with secondary dentition
Cosmetic appearance

Micrognathia occurs as part of the Pierre Robin syndrome.

Aetiology of cleft lip and palate
Idiopathic
Polygenic
Maternal drugs e.g. steroids, phenytoin
Environmental
Chromosomal e.g. Patau's syndrome
Pierre Robin syndrome

Treatment
It is current practice to undergo early lip closure between 0 and 3 months and often in the neonatal period. The palate is closed subsequently

between 6 and 12 months. Grommets are usually required. The advice of a speech therapist is essential early on to help with feeding and later with the development of speech.

Pierre Robin syndrome
This occurs in 1 in 30,000 live births. Features are
• micrognathia due to mandibular dysplasia
• midline cleft palate or high arched palate
• glossoptosis (causing pseudomacroglossia).
The most serious and potentially life-threatening problem in children with Pierre Robin syndrome is apnoea due to upper airway obstruction. The mandibular profile improves with age.

39. EPIGLOTTITIS AND CROUP   Answer: ADE

Factors that suggest epiglottitis rather than croup
Short history
High pyrexia with toxaemia
Absence of cough
Drooling
Neck extension

Factors that suggest croup rather then epiglottitis
Several days' history
Low grade pyrexia without toxaemia
Barking cough
Absence of drooling

Acute epiglottitis
This life-threatening condition is caused by *Haemophilus influenzae* type B. Peak age 6 months to 6 years. HIB immunisation has dramatically reduced the incidence. Treatment involves protection of the airway combined with high dose antibiotic therapy.

Croup
Croup (acute laryngotracheobronchitis) is caused by a number of viruses including para-influenza, influenza, respiratory syncitial virus and rhinovirus. The peak age is 6 months to 4 years. A number of patients have recurrent attacks.

Bacterial tracheitis
Bacterial tracheitis (pseudomembraneous croup) runs a more prolonged course. It usually occurs in children under 3 years of age. The presenting

features are of a barking cough associated with severe toxaemia and the absence of drooling. Causative organisms include *Staphylococcus aureus* and *Streptococcus pneumoniae*. High dose antibiotics are required and up to 80% of patients need intubation and ventilation.

40. MANAGEMENT OF ASTHMA   Answer: AB

It is essential to have a good knowledge of asthma management for the exam and to be clear about what devices should be used in children of different ages.

The aim of asthma management is to reduce the number of acute attacks and to prevent chronic symptoms. This is achieved by general measures (patients education, allergen avoidance and exercise prophylaxis) and drug therapy. Drug therapy is preventative and to control acute symptoms.

Acute attacks are principally treated with inhaled or nebulised broncho-dilators and oral steroids. Other therapies used in severe attacks include ipratropium bromide, intravenous aminophylline and intravenous salbutamol. Prophylactic agents include sodium cromoglycate and inhaled steroids. It is principally the latter which are used in children.

The device used to administer the drug is important. There are many different devices and it is appropriate for the candidate to be familiar with them all. In general a spacer device with a face mask or a nebuliser is used under the age of two and a spacer device without a face mask in older children. The oral route is not recommended. Devices like the turbohaler, dischaler, autohaler and rotahaler are best used in the over fives.

41. PRIMARY CILIARY DYSKINESIA   Answer: ABCE

This is an autosomal recessive group of disorders, the most common being Kartagener's syndrome. The incidence of primary ciliary dyskinesia is 1 in 16,000 live births.

Clinical features
Chronic bronchiectasis
Nasal polyposis
Recurrent sinusitis
Recurrent otitis media
Infertility, subfertility

Diagnosis
Saccharin test which assesses mucociliary clearance.
Light or phase contrast microscopy of scraping from the nasal mucosa.
Electron microscopic examination of cilia obtained from the nasal turbinates or tracheobronchial tree.

Treatment
Normal saline nebulisers
Bronchodilators
Mucolytics such as acetylcysteine
Physiotherapy
Regular antibiotics
Immunisation
Avoidance of cigarette smoke

Complications
Pneumothorax
Haemoptysis
Failure to thrive
Male infertility
Respiratory failure

A normal lifespan is possible if appropriately treated. Symptoms tend to improve after adolescence.

The classical Kartagener's syndrome is present in 50% of children with primary ciliary dyskinesia. Kartagener's syndrome includes:
• Chronic sinusitis
• Bronchiectasis
• Visceral situs inversus

42. CYSTIC FIBROSIS   Answer: ABD

Causes of clubbing
Congenital
Cyanotic congenital heart disease
Cystic fibrosis
Bronchiectasis, lung abscess, empyema
Inflammatory bowel disease
Cirrhosis, chronic active hepatitis

Cystic fibrosis
Inheritance of cystic fibrosis is autososmal recessive. Incidence of the carrier state is 1 in 20 and incidence of the disease 1 in 2500 in the United Kingdom. The gene locus is on chromosome 7.

10–15% present with meconium ileus. Meconium ileus can occur in children without cystic fibrosis.

10% of children with cystic fibrosis have no gastrointestinal involvement.

99% of males are infertile.

50% of children with cystic fibrosis have recurrent wheeze.

A thorough knowledge of the clinical features, genetic aspects and management of cystic fibrosis will be required for the exam.

43. BRONCHIECTASIS   Answer: BCDE

This is defined as persistent dilation of the bronchi, resulting from inflammatory destruction of its walls, associated with chronic cough with sputum production. It is characterised by periods of relapse and remission and poor weight gain is often a feature. Clubbing is a common finding. The commonest cause is cystic fibrosis. Contrast enhanced CT scanning is useful for diagnosis.

Other causes of bronchiectasis
Immunodeficiency
Alpha one antitrypsin deficiency
Primary ciliary dyskinesia
Foreign body
Lobar sequestration
Previous infection – measles, pertussis, pneumonia
Asthma

The management is with antibiotics and physiotherapy. Surgery is occasionally required if a defined lobe is affected and the patient unresponsive to medical treatment.

44. OBSTRUCTIVE SLEEP APNOEA   Answer: ABCE

Hypoventilation occurs resulting in hypoxia and hypercarbia (type II respiratory failure). This occurs until the central arousal mechanism operates and stimulates breathing by hypoxia. A definition of obstructive sleep apnoea has been offered which is 30 apnoeic episodes of 10 seconds or longer in a 7 hour period which occur secondary to airway obstruction.

The peak age is 2–6 years, with equal incidence in boys and girls. About 1% of snoring children have obstructive sleep apnoea. About 10% of children snore.

The symptoms and signs that occur as a consequence of nocturnal hypoxia and hypercapnia include:
- Apnoea
- Failure to thrive
- Excessive day time sleepiness
- Behavioural problems
- Polycythaemia
- Right ventricular hypertrophy
- Pulmonary hypertension

The diagnosis is made by clinical assessment and by overnight monitoring of respiratory rate, heart rate and oxygen saturations.

The treatment is with adenotonsillectomy and not just adenoidectomy. Tracheostomy is occasionally required.

Obstructive sleep apnoea is associated with active sleep. Nocturnal enuresis is common.

There is an increased risk of obstructive sleep apnoea in children with:
- Down's syndrome
- hypotonia from any cause
- developmental delay
- craniofacial anomalies
- sickle cell disease
- obesity.

45. *MYCOPLASMA PNEUMONIAE*   Answer: ABC

Mycoplasma pneumoniae is a bacteria without a cell wall. It is spread by droplet and humans are the only host. Incubation period 3 weeks.

The commonest clinical manifestation of infection is an atypical pneumonia presenting with cough. Infection is usually preceded by headache and sore throat. Wheeze is common. The chest X-ray appearance is usually worse than the symptoms and signs suggest. Peak incidence is in school age children.

Diagnosis is by serology with a positive *Mycoplasma* IgM in the acute illness and a convalescent rise in the *Mycoplasma* IgG titre. Culture is difficult. Cold agglutinins will be positive in 50%. White cell count is often normal.

Treatment is with erythromycin, bronchodilators and physiotherapy. Azithromycin and clarithromycin are other appropriate antibiotics. Tetracyclines can be given in adolescence.

Associations and complications of *Mycoplasma* infection

Skin	Erythema multiforme
	Stevens-Johnson syndrome
CNS	Meningoencephalitis
	Aseptic meningitis
	Cerebellar ataxia
	Guillain-Barre syndrome
Joints	Monoarticular arthritis
Cardiac	Myocarditis
	Pericarditis
Blood	Haemolysis
	Thrombocytopenia
Gut	Hepatitis
	Pancreatitis
	Protein-losing enteropathy

46. ACUTE TONSILLITIS   Answer: CE

Acute tonsillitis is rare in infancy. The peak incidence is around the age of 5. There is a second peak in adolescence.

Viral infections are much commoner then bacterial. The commonest viral agent is the adenovirus. Others include influenza, parainfluenza, RSV and adenovirus. The commonest bacteria is Group A beta haemolytic *Streptococcus*. Other agents include *Pneumococcus*, *Haemophilus* and *Mycoplasma*.

Tonsillar hypertrophy with exudate does not help to distinguish between a bacterial or a viral aetiology.

The differential diagnosis of tonsillitis includes diphtheria, agranulocytosis and infectious mononucleosis.

The indications for tonsillectomy are controversial but are often asked.
* Recurrent tonsillitis associated with failure to thrive and frequent school absence
* Quinsy
* Sleep apnoea
* To exclude a tonsillar tumour

The complications of tonsillectomy include haemorrhage. This can be either primary (within a few hours) or secondary (within a few days). Secondary haemorrhage is usually due to infection of the tonsillar bed and resolves once the infection is treated.

47. ANAPHYLAXIS   Answer: BCDE

Anaphylaxis is a type I immediate hypersensitivity reaction. It is IgE mediated. Anaphylaxis implies that the reaction is severe and involves difficulty in breathing, hypotension and shock. Untreated it can be fatal.

Management of anaphylaxis
Establish airway patency, high flow oxygen.
Adrenaline 10 μg/kg i.v. or i.m., 100 μg/kg via endotracheal tube.
Hydrocortisone 4 mg/kg i.v.
Chlorpheniramine 0.2 mg/kg i.v.
Repeat adrenaline every 15 minutes until sustained response seen. An infusion may need to be given.

Colloid 20 ml/kg.
If bronchospasm is severe then salbutamol can be given.

48. PULMONARY TUBERCULOSIS   Answer: BC

Mycobacterium tuberculosis is a Gram-positive acid-fast bacillus which turns red when stained with the Ziehl Nielson stain and is difficult to culture.

The reservoir for infection is the mammalian host (unlike atypical mycobacteria). Children are not normally infectious. Infectivity is highest in adults with cavitating open lung lesions.

The clinical features of infection are very variable and depend on the balance between bacterial multiplication and host response. Symptoms can either be from a primary complex or as a consequence of reactivation. The primary complex is a peripheral lung lesion (Ghon focus) with associated hilar lymphadenopathy.

The diagnosis of tuberculosis in childhood is difficult. Sputum is difficult to obtain and is rarely positive to acid-fast bacilli. Pointers include the clinical picture, history of contact, suggestive radiology and a positive tuberculin test. A positive mycobacterial culture may not be available and usually takes 6 weeks although it is diagnostic. Bronchoscopy with lung biopsy is sometimes required. Recent work has been done using the polymerase chain reaction to identify mycobacterial DNA.

Tuberculin testing is best done using the Mantoux test. This is often difficult to interpret. It can be negative in fulminating disease in its early stages and in children with HIV infection. In addition a cohort of children will have been given BCG. A strongly positive Mantoux (>15 mm induration in response to 0.1 ml of 1 in 1000 preparation) is suggestive of infection even if BCG has previously been given.

Treatment is with isoniazid, rifampicin (6 months) and pyrazinamide (2 months).

Side effects of antituberculous therapy
Isoniazid: peripheral neuropathy (preventable with pyridoxine), skin rashes, abnormal liver function tests
Rifampicin: skin rashes, abnormal LFTs

Pyrazinamide: skin rashes, abnormal LFTs, photosensitivity
Ethambutol: ocular toxicity
Streptomycin: ototoxicity, nephrotoxicity

49. LUNG DEVELOPMENT   Answer: CD

Lung development is divided into four stages according to microscopic appearance.

Embryonic
0–7 weeks. Lung foundation is laid down. Lung bud develops as a ventral diverticulum of the foregut (endodermal). Surrounding mesenchyme also derived from the foregut. All segmental bronchi are developed by the end of the embryonic phase.

Pseudoglandular
7–17 weeks. Conducting airways are developed with continuous branching of bronchial buds. Adult number of airways proximal to the acini are present by the 16th week of gestation. Epithelial lining differentiates. Goblet and serous cells are identifiable by 16 weeks. All pre acinar vessels are present by 17 weeks.

Canalicular
17–26 weeks. This phase sees the maturing of the conducting airways and the development of the terminal respiratory units. There is an increase in size of the proximal airways with an increase in cartilage, muscle and glandular tissue. By 22 weeks type I and type II pneumocytes are seen.

Alveolar
27 weeks to term. This period sees the further development of gas exchange units such that by term one-third to a half of the adult number of alveoli are present. Pre acinar airways increase in size and there is a continued increase in the number of goblet cells.

The acinus is a functional unit comprising alveoli, alveolar ducts and respiratory bronchioles.

Alveoli increase in number up until 4–8 years of age.

50. PEAK EXPIRATORY FLOW RATE   Answer: DE

The peak expiratory flow rate is the maximum expiratory flow rate following a full inspiration. It is dependent upon the diameter of the airways at the narrowest point and the intrathoracic pressure generated.

It is effort dependent. Very few children under the age of 5 years can do a peak flow.

Forced expiratory volume

The FEV_1 is the volume of air that can be forcibly expired in one second. It is less effort dependent and more reproducible than the peak expiratory flow rate. In asthma the residual volume will increase reducing the forced vital capacity.

51. HYDROLYSED PROTEIN FORMULA   Answer: AD

A hydrolysed protein is one which is broken down into oligopeptides and peptides. A hydrolysed protein milk formula is therefore one which does not contain whole protein. An elemental formula is one in which the protein is broken down into amino acids.

The following are hydrolysed protein formulae:
• Pregestimil
• Nutramigen
• Prejomin
• Pepti-Junior
• Flexical

Neocate is an elemental formula.

These formulae are indicated in conditions where the protein in milk is implicated in the pathogenesis as an antigen. Examples include:
• Cows' milk protein intolerance
• Post gastroenteritis
• Severe eczema

Hydrolysed protein formulae are generally lactose free as are soya milk preparations. Wysoy and Formula S are both lactose-free soya milks.

The indications for a soya milk preparation are similar to the indications for a hydrolysate. A soya preparation is cheaper. If used for cows' milk protein intolerance then cross reactivity with soya protein is common and about one-sixth of patients will also be intolerant to the soya preparation. In this circumstance it is necessary to use a hydrolysed formula.

Prematil is a preterm formula. Maxijul is a glucose polymer.

52. MECKEL'S DIVERTICULUM   Answer: ABDE

Meckel's diverticulum is a remnant of the vitello-intestinal duct which is present in 2% of individuals. 50% contain ectopic gastric, pancreatic or colonic tissue.

It is located in the distal ileum on the anti-mesenteric border within 100 cm of the ileo-caecal valve and is around 5–6 cm long.

It usually presents with intermittent, painless blood per rectum. Bleeding can be quite severe and may require a blood transfusion. Other presentations include intussusception (commoner in older males), perforation and peritonitis.

The technetium scan is used to look for ectopic gastric mucosa.

Other causes of blood per rectum in childhood
Anal fissure
Volvulus
Intussusception
Peptic ulcer
Polyp
Inflammatory bowel disease
Haemolytic uraemic syndrome
Infective colitis
Henoch-Schoenlein purpura
Vascular malformation
Oesophagitis/varices
Epistaxis
Necrotising enterocolitis

Polyposis in childhood
Juvenile polyps
85% of polyps seen in childhood. Present at age 2–6 years with painless blood per rectum. Not premalignant.

Peutz-Jeghers syndrome
Autosomal dominantly inherited. Diffuse gastrointestinal hamartomatous polyps associated with hyperpigmentation of the buccal mucosa and lips. Premalignant.

Gardener's syndrome
Familial adenomatous polyposis coli
Best considered together. Both conditions are inherited as autosomal dominant. Gardener's syndrome is familial adenomatous polyposis plus bony lesions, subcutaneous tumours and cysts. Both conditions carry a very high risk of colonic carcinoma and prophylactic colectomy at the end of the second decade is advised.

53. BREAST FEEDING   Answer: AE

This is a difficult question which recurs and is somewhat controversial. Contraindications to breast feeding are either absolute (always apply) or relative.

Absolute contraindications
Galactosaemia
Cytotoxic (immunosuppressive) drugs e.g. methotrexate, cyclophosphamide

Relative contraindications
Tuberculosis
Hepatitis B
Chickenpox
Maternal ill health
Amiodarone
Atenolol
Ergot alkaloids
Gold salts
Radiopharmaceuticals

With regard to tuberculosis, infants can be immunised at birth with isoniazid resistant BCG and treated with a course of isoniazid.

With regard to HIV, the virus has been cultured from breast milk and is transmitted in it. In the Western world this makes breast feeding contraindicated as it will increase the perinatal transmission rate. The problem is not so straightforward in the developing world where the risks associated with bottle feeding are high.

54. ABETALIPOPROTEINAEMIA   Answer: ADE

The inheritance is autosomally recessive.

Long chain fatty acids are transmitted as chylomicrons along the thoracic duct. Betalipoprotein is part of the chylomicron. The pathogenesis of abetalipoproteinaemia is failure of chylomicron formation with impaired absorption of long chain fats with fat retention in the enterocyte.

Fat malabsorption occurs from birth. The condition presents in early infancy with failure to thrive, abdominal distension and foul smelling, bulky stools. Symptoms of vitamin E deficiency (ataxia, peripheral neuropathy and retinitis pigmentosa) develop later. The child is normal at birth.

Laboratory diagnosis:
- Low serum cholesterol
- Very low plasma triglyceride level
- Acanthocytes on examination of the peripheral blood film
- Absence of betalipoprotein in the plasma

Treatment is by substituting medium chain triglycerides for long chain triglycerides in the diet. Medium chain triglycerides are absorbed via the portal vein rather than the thoracic duct. In addition, high doses of the fat-soluble vitamins (A, D, E and K) are required. Most of the neurological abnormalities are reversible if high doses of vitamin E are given early.

Causes of acanthocytosis
Abetalipoproteinaemia
Chronic liver disease
Hyposplenism

Associations of retinitis pigmentosa
Abetalipoproteinaemia
Laurence-Moon-Biedl syndrome
Usher's syndrome
Refsum's disease
Alport's syndrome
Familial
Idiopathic

55. ACRODERMATITIS ENTEROPATHICA　　　Answer: CDE

This shows autosomal recessive inheritance. The basic defect is impaired absorption of zinc in the gut.

It presents with skin rash around the mouth and perianal area, chronic diarrhoea at the time of weaning and recurrent infections. The hair has a reddish tint, alopecia is characteristic. Superinfection with *Candida* is common as are paronychia, dystrophic nails, poor wound healing and ocular changes (photophobia, blepharitis, corneal dystrophy).

Diagnosis is by serum zinc levels and the constellation of clinical signs.

This is difficult as the serum zinc is low as part of the acute phase response. Measurement of white cell zinc levels is more accurate. The plasma metallothionein level can also be measured. Metallothionein is a zinc binding protein that is decreased in zinc deficiency but not in the acute phase response.

The condition responds very well to treatment with oral zinc.

Zinc deficiency can cause the following:
Iron deficiency anaemia
Acrodermatitis enteropathica
Hyperpigmentation
Poor wound healing
Immunodeficiency
Growth failure
Hypogonadism

Clinically important trace elements
Chromium
Copper
Cobalt
Molybdenum
Manganese
Selenium
Zinc

56. VITAMIN A   Answer: ABCDE

Vitamin A is a fat soluble vitamin (as are D, E and K). Deficiency causes night blindness, poor growth, xerophthalmia, follicular hyperplasia and impaired resistance to infection.

Excess causes carotenaemia, hyperostosis with bone pain, hepatomegaly, alopecia and desquamation of the palms. Acute intoxication causes raised intracranial pressure.

Dietary sources are
• milk
• fat
• fruit and vegetables
• egg
• liver

Vitamin A has an important role in the resistance to infection particularly at mucosal surfaces. In the Third World where vitamin A deficiency is endemic, vitamin A reduces the morbidity and mortality in severe measles.

57. BREAST FEEDING   Answer: ABD

Breast feeding and infection
10% of the protein in mature breast milk is secretory IgA. Lymphocytes, macrophages, proteins with non-specific anti-bacterial activity and complement are also present. There have been many studies in the Third World to show that infants fed formula milk have a higher mortality and morbidity, particularly from gastrointestinal infection.

In the UK, studies have been done which show:
- Breast feeding for more than 13 weeks reduces the incidence of gastrointestinal and respiratory infections.
- The response to immunisation with the HIB vaccine is higher in breast fed than in formula fed infants.
- The risk of necrotising enterocolitis in low birth weight babies is lower in those who are breast fed.

Breast feeding and allergy
The incidence of atopic eczema in infants born to atopic mothers is reduced by breast feeding. Overall however there is no reduction in atopy apart from this specific circumstance.

Breast feeding and neurological development
Although there are confounding variables which make study of this subject difficult, there is work that suggests that neurological development is enhanced in breast fed infants. I doubt however that an MCQ would be set on this controversial point.

Breast feeding and diabetes
Infants who are breast fed have a reduced risk of developing diabetes.

Breast feeding and infantile colic
There is no good evidence to show that breast feeding reduces the incidence of infantile colic.

58. VITAMIN K   Answer: CDE

British Paediatric Association guidelines on vitamin K prophylaxis for haemorrhagic disease of the newborn:
- All newborn infants should be given vitamin K.
- Intramuscular vitamin K, 1 mg, ensures adequate prophylaxis in normal term infants.
- One dose of 1 mg vitamin K orally is adequate prophylaxis for the majority of normal term infants. Further doses should be considered for breast fed infants.
- Infants with jaundice suggestive of cholestasis, and infants with unexplained bleeding, should receive further vitamin K, preferably parenterally.

Vitamin K is a fat soluble vitamin, which is contained in cows' milk, green leafy vegetables and pork. There is very little in breast milk.

Deficiency in the newborn period presents as haemorrhagic disease of the newborn. This usually presents on day 2 or 3 with bleeding from the umbilical stump, haematemesis and malaena, epistaxis or excessive bleeding from puncture sites. Diagnosis is by prolongation of the prothrombin and partial thromboplastin times with the thrombin time and fibrinogen levels being normal. Treatment is with fresh frozen plasma and vitamin K.

There is no proven association between intramuscular vitamin K and childhood cancer.

59. XYLOSE TOLERANCE TEST   Answer: BDE

Xylose tolerance test
The xylose tolerance test is an indirect method used to assess small bowel absorption. Xylose is a carbohydrate. A load (15 mg/m^2, max 25 g) is ingested and a blood level taken at 1 hour. A level of less than 25 mg/dl is suggestive of carbohydrate malabsorption. The test is neither sensitive nor specific. False-positive results are obtained in pernicious anaemia and when there is gut oedema.

Other indirect tests of gastrointestinal function
Serum albumin
Faecal fat
Stool pH and reducing substances

Stool alpha 1 antitrypsin
Hydrogen breath test

Hydrogen breath test
The hydrogen breath test looks for carbohydrate malabsorption. The principle is that malabsorbed carbohydrate will pass to the colon where it is metabolised by bacteria and hydrogen gas is released. The gas is then absorbed and released in the breath. If there is a peak it suggests carbohydrate malabsorption. An early peak raises the possibility of bacterial overgrowth. Lactulose which is a non-absorbable carbohydrate can be given to ensure the colonic flora can metabolise carbohydrate and to assess transit time.

Albumin
Hypoalbuminaemia can occur secondary to reduced protein intake, reduced production by the liver in chronic liver disease, gut and renal loss.

Alpha-1 antitrypsin in the stool is a sensitive marker of enteric protein loss.

Gastrointestinal causes of protein loss
Inflammatory bowel disease
Coeliac disease
Cystic fibrosis
Schwachman syndrome
Infection
Intestinal lymphangiectasia
Mentriere's disease

60. FOLIC ACID (FOLATE)   Answer: AC

Dietary sources of folate include liver, green vegetables, cereals, orange, milk, yeast and mushrooms. It is destroyed by excessive cooking. It is absorbed from the proximal small bowel.

Deficiency causes megaloblastic anaemia, irritability, poor weight gain and chronic diarrhoea. Thrombocytopenia can occur.

The serum folate reflects recent changes in folate status and the red cell folate is an indicator of the total body stores. Treatment of deficiency is with oral folic acid. Folate levels are not affected by the acute phase response.

Causes of folate deficiency
Reduced intake
Coeliac disease
Tropical sprue
Blind loop syndrome
Congenital folate malabsorption (autosomal recessive)
Increased requirements (infancy, pregnancy, exfoliative skin disease)
Increased loss (haemodialysis)
Methotrexate
Trimethoprim
Anticonvulsants
Oral contraceptive pill

There is an association between folate deficiency in early pregnancy and neural tube defects in the fetus.

61. BREAST MILK   Answer: BCDE

The composition of human milk at term per 100 ml
(Department of Health 1988)

Energy	70 kcal
Protein	1.3 g
Carbohydrate	7.0 g
Fat	4.2 g
Osmolality	264 mosm/kg
Sodium	0.65 mmol
Potassium chloride	1.54 mmol
Calcium	0.88 mmol
Magnesium	0.12 mmol
Phosphate	0.48 mmol
Iron	1.36 micromol

62. CARBOHYDRATE INTOLERANCE IN   Answer: BC
CHILDHOOD

Disorders of disaccharide absorption
Primary
  Congenital alactasia
  Congenital lactose intolerance
  Sucrose–isomaltase deficiency

Secondary (acquired)
   Post enteritis (rotavirus), neonatal surgery, malnutrition
   Late onset lactose intolerance

Disorders of monosaccharide absorption
Primary
   Glucose–galactose malabsorption
Secondary (acquired)
   Post enteritis, neonatal surgery, malnutrition

Carbohydrate intolerance is usually lactose intolerance and usually acquired. The deficient enzyme is the brush border enzyme lactase which hydrolyses lactose into glucose and galactose. The intolerance will present with characteristic loose explosive stools. The diagnosis is made by looking for reducing substance in the stool following carbohydrate ingestion. The test used is the Clinitest tablets (which detect reducing substance in the stool) and the detection of more than 0.5% is significant. Treatment is with a lactose free formula in infancy and a reduced lactose intake in later childhood.

Following gastroenteritis, carbohydrate intolerance can be either to disaccharides or monosaccharides. Both types of intolerance are usually transient and both respond to removal of the offending carbohydrate. Both mono- and disaccharides will result in the reducing substances in the stool being positive.

Glucose-galactose malabsorption
This is a rare autosomal recessively inherited condition characterised by rapid onset watery diarrhoea from birth. This responds to witholding glucose (stopping feeds) and relapses on reintroduction. The diagnosis is essentially a clinical one. Reducing substances in the stool will be positive and small bowel biopsy and dissacharide estimation normal. Treatment is by using fructose as the main carbohydrate source. Fructose is absorbed by a different mechanism to glucose and galactose.

63. PRETERM AND TERM FORMULA   **Answer: ACD**

The principal differences are that preterm formula contains more electrolytes, calories and minerals. All of the following are higher in preterm than term formula: Energy, protein, carbohydrate, fat, osmolality, sodium, potassium, calcium, magnesium, phosphate and iron. There are many different formula feeds on the market and it is important to be aware of the differences between mature breast milk, term and preterm formula and cows' milk.

64. HUMAN (BREAST) MILK AND COWS' MILK
Answer: None correct

The energy content is the same. Human milk contains less protein than cows' milk – the cows' milk having a much higher casein content. The fat, although different qualitatively is the same in amount. Human milk contains more carbohydrate. Cows' milk contains more of all of the minerals except iron and copper.

65. NUTRITIONAL SUPPLEMENTS
Answer: AD

Nutritional supplements based on glucose polymer
Maxijul
Caloreen
Polycal
Fortical
Hycal

Nutritional supplements based on fat
Calogen
Liquigen
MCT Pepdite

Nutritional supplements based on glucose polymer and fat
Duocal

Fat based nutritional supplements generally contain more calories per ml. Calogen contains 450 kcal per 100 g and Maxijul between 180 and 380 kcal per 100 g depending on the preparation used.

Term formula milks, either whey or casein based contain the same amount of calories, which is the same as mature breast milk and cows' milk (66–70 kcal per 100 ml).

Breast milk fortifiers are often added to breast milk given to preterm babies.

66. IMMUNOGLOBULIN A   Answer: BDE

IgA makes up 15% of circulating immunoglobulin. In its secretory form it is the predominant immunoglobulin at respiratory and gastrointestinal surfaces.

Selective IgA deficiency
This is a common disorder, with an incidence of 1 in 600. It is associated with an increased incidence of infection, atopic disease and rheumatic disorders.
*   Respiratory tract infection
*   Gastrointestinal tract infection, particularly giardiasis
*   Crohn's disease, ulcerative colitis, coeliac disease
*   Autoimmune/rheumatoid conditions including rheumatoid arthritis, systemic lupus erythematosus and pernicious anaemia

Immunoglobulin therapy is not worthwhile if isolated IgA deficiency is present. This is because there is only a small amount of IgA in immunoglobulin preparations and sensitisation is therefore likely. If there is coexistent IgG deficiency or IgG subclass deficiency then immunoglobulin therapy may be appropriate.

67. FAILURE TO THRIVE   Answer: CD

Failure to thrive is a failure to gain weight at an adequate rate. The aetiology can be organic or non-organic (psychosocial deprivation). Low birth weight and preterm birth are associations of failure to thrive but not causes of it.

Failure to thrive occurs as a consequence of one of the following:
*   Failure of carer to offer adequate calories
*   Failure of the child to take sufficient calories
*   Failure of the child to retain adequate calories.

Clearly this can be organic or non-organic. Insufficient calories may be offered as a consequence of parental neglect or because of a failure of the carer to appreciate the calorie requirements of the child. Insufficient calories may be taken as a consequence of feeding difficulties (for example cerebral palsy) and calories may not be retained because of absorptive defects or lost because of vomiting or diarrhoea.

The investigation of failure to thrive is generally only fruitful wh specific pointers to organic problems are elucidated in the history.

The management of non-organic failure to thrive requires dietary assessment often accompanied by hospital admission for evaluation and to ensure an adequate weight gain can be obtained if sufficient calories are given.

Organic causes of failure to thrive

Gastrointestinal	Coeliac disease, cows' milk protein intolerance, gastro-oesophageal reflux
Renal	Urinary tract infection, renal tubular acidosis
Cardiopulmonary	Cardiac disease, bronchopulmonary dysplasia
Endocrine	Hypothyroidism
Neurological	Cerebral palsy
Infection/Immunodeficiency	HIV, malignancy
Metabolic	Inborn errors of metabolism
Congenital	Chromosomal abnormalities
ENT	Adenotonsillar hypertrophy

68. CARBOHYDRATE DIGESTION   Answer: ABD

Carbohydrates are consumed as monosaccharides (glucose, fructose, galactose), disaccharides (lactose, sucrose, maltose, isomaltose) and polysaccharides (starch, dextrins, glycogen).

Salivary and pancreatic amylase breaks starch down into oligo-saccharides and disaccharides. Pancreatic amylase aids carbohydrate digestion but carbohydrate digestion is not dependent on it.

Disaccharidases (maltase, sucrase, lactase) in the microvilli hydrolyse
- oligo- and disaccharides into monosaccharides
- maltose into glucose
- isomaltose into glucose
- sucrose into glucose and fructose
- lactose into glucose and galactose

Monosaccharides are then absorbed, glucose and galactose by an active transport mechanism and fructose by facilitated diffusion.

69. WILSON'S DISEASE (HEPATOLENTICULAR DEGENERATION)   Answer: BDE

- Incidence 1 in 500,000.
- Autosomal recessive inheritance.
- Gene known and is on chromosome 13.

The pathology is a consequence of decreased biliary excretion of copper and impaired caeruloplasmin production. Caeruloplasmin is the plasma protein which transports copper.

Effects of Wilson's Disease

Liver: Chronic active hepatitis, portal hypertension and fulminant hepatic failure

Brain: Progressive lenticular degeneration due to copper deposition

Cornea: Kayser-Fleischer rings

Lens: Sunflower cataract

Kidney: Renal tubular disorders

Blood: Haemolysis

The hepatic presentation can be as asymptomatic hepatomegaly, acute hepatitis, chronic active hepatitis, portal hypertension (ascites, oedema, variceal haemorrhage) or fulminant hepatic failure. The lenticular degeneration usually presents with tremor.

Diagnosis is by a low plasma caeruloplasmin level and high urinary copper excretion. The latter can occur in other forms of hepatitis and a liver biopsy is often required. In equivocal cases the increased copper excretion after chelation with D-penicillamine is of diagnostic importance. Serum copper levels are not helpful.

Untreated the condition is fatal. Treated the prognosis is good. Treatment is with oral penicillamine as a copper binding agent in conjunction with a low copper diet. Patients on penicillamine require vitamin B6 supplements as it is an antimetabolite.

The condition does not usually present under the age of 5 years.

70. NEONATAL JAUNDICE   Answer: BCE

Neonatal jaundice is classified as either early (<14 days) or late (>14 days). Jaundice can either be conjugated (direct) or unconjugated (indirect). Unconjugated is fat soluble and does not spill over into the urine. Conjugated is water soluble and is present in the urine as bilirubinuria.

Up to 50% of normal newborns become clinically jaundiced in the early neonatal period.

Causes of unconjugated hyperbilirubinaemia in the neonatal period
Physiological
Breast milk
Infection
Haemolysis
    Rhesus incompatibility
    ABO incompatibility
    Hereditary spherocytosis
    Glucose 6 phosphate dehydrogenase deficiency
Polycythaemia
Hypothyroidism
Galactosaemia
Pyloric stenosis

71. FLAT SMALL INTESTINAL MUCOSA   Answer: ACE

Causes
Coeliac disease
Transient gluten intolerance
Cows' milk sensitive enteropathy
Soy protein intolerance
Gastroenteritis and post gastroenteritis syndromes
Giardiasis
Auto-immune enteropathy
Acquired hypogammaglobulinaemia
Tropical sprue
Protein energy malnutrition
Severe combined immunodeficiency
Anti-neoplastic therapy

Coeliac disease

- Prevalence is 1 in 2000.
- Associations are with HLA B8, DR7, DR3 and DQw2.
- There is an increased incidence in first degree relatives.
- Intolerance is to gluten which is present in wheat, rye, barley and oats.

Coeliac disease presents after 6 months of age (i.e. after gluten has been introduced into the diet). Chronic diarrhoea and poor weight gain (short stature in older children) generally occur. Other features include anorexia, lethargy, generalised irritability, abdominal distension and pallor.

Diagnosis is by small bowel biopsy (endoscopic duodenal or jejunal). The characteristic features on biopsy are of sub-total villous atrophy, crypt hypertrophy, intracellular lymphocytes and a lamina propria plasma cell infiltrate. It is of crucial importance that the child's gluten intake is adequate at the time of the biopsy.

Treatment is with a gluten free diet for life. There is a long term risk of small bowel lymphoma if the diet is not adhered to. The gluten free diet itself has no long term complications.

The standards for the diagnosis of coeliac disease are set out by the European Society of Paediatric Gastroenterology. Diagnosis is confirmed by characteristic histology and a clinical remission on a gluten free diet. There are indications for a subsequent gluten challenge and these include initial diagnostic uncertainty and when the diagnosis is made under the age of 2 years. The latter being because at that age there are other causes of a flat jejunal biopsy and these are listed above. A gluten challenge involves an initial control biopsy on a gluten free diet followed by a period on gluten with a repeat biopsy after 3–6 months and then again after 2 years, sooner if symptoms develop. There are reports of late relapse following gluten challenge.

Antibody testing in the screening of children with failure to thrive and in the ongoing management of children with coeliac disease is helpful. The biopsy remains the gold standard for diagnosis.

Antibody tests available
Ig G anti-gliadin
IgA anti-gliadin
IgA anti-reticulin
IgA anti-endomysial

The IgA anti-endomysial antibody is the most sensitive and specific.

Associations of coeliac disease
Increased incidence of small bowel malignancy, especially lymphoma
Increased incidence of IgA deficiency
Increased incidence of autoimmune thyroid disease, pernicious anaemia
and diabetes mellitus (HLA B8 associations)
Dermatitis herpetiformis

72. HEPATITIS   Answer: A

Hepatitis B
This is a DNA virus. Diagnosis is by detection of the HBsAg. HBeAg
positive patients carry a larger virus load and are more infectious. Acute
and ongoing chronic infection is associated with anti HBcIgM. Anti Hbe
and anti HBs antibodies appear as an effective immune response
develops. All HBsAg positive subjects are infective. Transmission is
parenteral.

The perinatal transmission rate is dependent on the maternal serology. If
the mother is HBsAg positive and HBeAg negative the risk is 12–25%.
If the mother is HBsAg positive and HBeAg positive the risk is 90%.

The younger the age at infection the less the likelihood of symptomatic
liver disease but the greater the risk of prolonged viral carriage. 90% of
infants infected in the first year of life become chronic carriers.

Clinically the disease is often asymptomatic but an acute hepatic picture
can develop. Acute liver failure occurs in less than 1%. The risk of
fulminant hepatitis is increased by co-infection with hepatitis D. In those
with a typical hepatic picture the chronic carrier rate is low.

Chronicity results in an increased risk of cirrhosis and hepatocellular
carcinoma. Males are more likely to become chronic carriers than
females. Chronically infected children have a 25% lifetime risk of
cirrhosis or hepatocellular carcinoma.

Prevention is by both active and passive immunisation.

Interferon alpha is a recognised treatment of chronic infection.

Hepatitis D
Hepatitis D is an RNA virus which requires the hepatitis B surface antigen for its assembly and virulence. It is transmitted like hepatitis B. The severity of the liver damage increases if there is coexistent hepatitis B infection. Diagnosis is by serology. Hepatitis B vaccine or immunity following infection offers protection.

73. HEPATITIS   Answer: BD

Hepatitis A
This is an RNA virus. Diagnosis is by detection of the hepatitis A virus IgM. Transmission is faeco-oral. There is no carrier state and fulminant hepatic failure is very rare (<0.1%). The liver function however may be abnormal for up to 1 year.

Prevention is by either passive or active immunisation. Passive immunisation is with immunoglobulin which lasts for 3–6 months. Active immunisation is with a live attenuated virus. Booster immunisation being required after 12–18 months.

Clinical symptoms are initially non-specific and include anorexia, nausea, fatigue and fever associated with epigastric pain and tender hepatomegaly. The icteric phase then develops with jaundice, pale stools and dark urine. Sometimes there is pruritus, depression and persistent jaundice with raised transaminases for a prolonged period. The prothrombin time should be monitored. A raised prothrombin time raises the possibility of severe hepatic necrosis or decompensation of underlying liver disease.

Hepatitis C
This is an RNA virus. Transmission is either perinatal or parenteral. Diagnosis is by serology. Blood for transfusion is routinely screened.

Infection can either be asymptomatic or an acute hepatitis can occur. Chronic infection is common with the development of cirrhosis and hepatocellular carcinoma in a number of cases. Treatment with interferon-alpha has been given. No vaccine is available.

Fulminant hepatitis is uncommon but can occur.

Hepatitis E

This is an RNA virus. Epidemics occur in developing countries. UK infection is usually in travellers from endemic areas. Transmission is faeco-oral.

The clinical course of hepatitis E infection is similar to hepatitis A. Complete recovery from acute infection occurs. Chronic infection has not been described although acute fulminant hepatic failure can occur and is more common during pregnancy.

Diagnosis is by serology. No vaccine treatment or prophylaxis is available.

74. COLITIS   Answer: BC

Abdominal pain associated with bloody diarrhoea is indicative of a colitis. Colitis can be infective or non-infective.

Causes of infective colitis
Salmonella species
Shigella species
Campylobacter pylori
E. coli 0157 (and other *E. coli*)
Clostridium difficile (pseudomembraneous colitis)
Yersinia
Tuberculosis
Cytomegalovirus
Entamoeba histolytica
Enterobius vermicularis

Causes of a non-infective colitis
Ulcerative colitis
Crohn's disease
Necrotising enterocolitis
Microscopic colitis
Behçet's disease
Food allergic colitis

75. *GIARDIA LAMBLIA*

Answer: BCE

This is a protozoal parasite which is infective in the cyst form. It also exists in the trophozoite form. It is found in contaminated food and water.

Clinical manifestations may be
- Asymptomatic
- Acute diarrhoeal disease
- Chronic diarrhoea

The latter may be associated with malabsorption and an abnormal small bowel mucosa.

Diagnosis is by stool examination for cysts or examination of the duodenal aspirate at small bowel biopsy. Treatment is with metronidazole.

76. INTUSSUSCEPTION

Answer: ADE

- Peak incidence aged 6–9 months
- 1–4 per 1000 live births
- Male to female ratio 4:1
- Commoner in the spring and autumn

Usually presents with spasmodic pain, pallor and irritability. Vomiting is an early feature and rapidly progresses to being bile stained. Passage of blood-stained stools often occurs and a mass is frequently palpable. The presentation however is often atypical.

The intussusception is usually ileo-caecal, the origin being either the ileo-caecal valve or the terminal ileum.

An identifiable cause is commoner in those who present later – Meckel's diverticulum, polyp, reduplication, lymphosarcoma and Henoch-Schoenlein purpura being examples.

Diagnosis is usually on clinical grounds. Confirmation is by plain abdominal X-ray, ultrasound or air or barium enema examination.

Treatment is either with air or barium enema reduction if the history is short or surgically at laparotomy. Resuscitation with albumin is usually required. Contraindications to barium enema include peritonitis and signs of perforation.

77. GILBERT'S SYNDROME   Answer: ADE

Gilbert's syndrome is defined as unconjugated hyperbilirubinaemia with no evidence of haemolysis and normal liver function tests. The liver biopsy is normal.

The prevalence is 6%. The condition is more common in males than females. Inheritance is autosomal dominant with incomplete expression.

The pathogenesis is unclear but probably represents a mild functional deficiency of the enzyme UDP glucuronyl transferase.

The clinical picture is of mild fluctuating jaundice (serum bilirubin 30–50 micromol/l) aggravated by infection, exertion and fasting. Of some diagnostic use, the condition improves with phenobarbitone and worsens with nicotinic acid.

Other inherited causes of hyperbilirubinaemia include:

Crigler Najjar syndrome
Type one (autosomal recessive) is due to complete absence of UDP glucuronyl transferase in the liver. Jaundice presents soon after birth and rapidly progresses to toxic levels (kernicterus). Untreated, death usually occurs by the end of the first year. Diagnosis is by estimation of hepatic UDP glucuronyl transferase activity in a specimen obtained by needle liver biopsy. Repeated exchange transfusions and phototherapy aid short term survival. The only long term therapeutic option is liver transplantation.
Type two (autosomal dominant) is less severe and responds to treatment with phenobarbitone. Kernicterus is unusual.

Dubin Johnson syndrome
Autosomal recessive. Presents with conjugated hyperbilirubinaemia and bilirubinuria. It is due to a reduced ability to transport organic anions such as bilirubin glucuronide into the biliary tree. There is black pigmentation of the liver on biopsy. Life expectancy is normal. Jaundice is exacerbated by alcohol, infection and pregnancy.

Rotor syndrome
Autosomal recessive. Presents with conjugated hyperbilirubinaemia. It is due to a deficiency in organic anion uptake as well as excretion. No black pigment in the liver. Normal life expectancy. Jaundice exacerbated by alcohol, infection and pregnancy. Sulphabromophthalein excretion test is abnormal.

78. ULCERATIVE COLITIS   Answer: ACDE

Ulcerative colitis is an inflammatory disease limited to the colonic and rectal mucosa. It is the more distal bowel that is the most involved. Inflammation is neither pan-enteric or transmural as is seen in Crohn's disease. A backwash ileitis into the terminal ileum is often seen. The characteristic histology in the colon is of mucosal and submucosal inflammation with goblet cell depletion, cryptitis and crypt abscesses but no granulomas. The inflammatory change is usually diffuse rather than patchy.

The aetiology is unknown. The disease is more common in females than in males. Childhood prevalence is around 4 per 100,000. 10–15% present in childhood.

Although unusual, the disease can present with predominantly extra-intestinal manifestations including growth failure, arthropathy, erythema nodosum, occult blood loss, non-specific abdominal pain, cholangitis and raised inflammatory indices.

The gut disease can be mild, moderate or severe. The symptoms of colitis are diarrhoea, blood per rectum and abdominal pain. Systemic disturbance can accompany the more severe disease; tachycardia, fever, weight loss, anaemia, hypoalbuminaemia and leucocytosis.

Complications of ulcerative colitis
Toxic megacolon
Growth failure
Cholangitis
Cancer
Non-malignant stricture

The cancer risk reflects the disease severity and duration of disease. Regular screening is carried out in adult life.

Diagnosis is by endoscopy and biopsy with the classical histological features being shown. A small number of children have an indeterminate or unclassified colitis. The differential diagnosis of colitis is wide and a list of the causes of a non-infective and an infective colitis are listed elsewhere.

Treatment of ulcerative colitis
5 ASA derivatives
Local or systemic steroids
Azathioprine to reduce steroid toxicity in steroid-dependent patients
Surgery

Differences between Crohn's disease and ulcerative colitis

Crohn's	Ulcerative colitis
Pan-enteric	Colon only
Skip lesions	Diffuse
Transmural	Mucosal
Granulomas	Crypt abscesses
Peri-anal disease	

79. RECURRENT ABDOMINAL PAIN

Answer: AC

Recurrent abdominal pain is very common in childhood affecting up to 10% of the school age population. In the majority of cases the aetiology is non-organic. The condition is more common in girls than in boys and a family history is common. The pain is usually peri-umbilical and rarely associated with other gastrointestinal symptoms such as diarrhoea, blood per rectum or weight loss.

Abdominal pain accompanied by other symptoms is suggestive of organic pathology. Night pain is suggestive of oesophagitis or peptic ulceration. Diarrhoea with blood per rectum suggests a colitis and diarrhoea associated with weight loss a malabsorption syndrome.

80. PORTAL HYPERTENSION

Answer: D

Aetiology

Pre Hepatic
Portal vein thrombosis
- sepsis
- pancreatitis
- umbilical catheterisation (artery or vein)
- omphalitis

Intra Hepatic
   Pre-sinusoidal
      - neoplasia
      - schistosomiasis
      - heptic cyst
   Sinusoidal
      - cirrhosis
      - biliary atresia
      - neonatal hepatitis
      - alpha-1 antitrypsin deficiency
   Post-sinusoidal
      - veno-occlusive disease

Post Hepatic
   Budd-Chiari syndrome
   Right ventricular failure
   Constrictive pericaditis

Clinical features of portal hypertension
Splenomegaly
Ascites
Prominent abdominal vessels (caput medusa)
Oesophageal varices
Haemorrhoids
Rectal varices

Complications of portal hypertension
Ascites – compromising respiration, infection, hypoalbuminaemia
Variceal bleeding
Porto-systemic encephalopathy
Splenomegaly with hypersplenism

81. HOMOCYSTINURIA AND MARFAN'S SYNDROME   Answer: CD

Homocystinuria

The incidence of homocystinuria is 1 in 300,000. Inheritance is autosomal recessive. Prenatal diagnosis is possible.

It is a disorder of the conversion of methionine into cystine with a consequent accumulation of homocystine.

Clinical features of homocystinuria

Normal at birth
Marfanoid features, tall and thin with long fingers, the lower segment of the body longer than the upper segment and an arm span greater than height.
Subluxed lens – downward and inward
Stiff joints
Connective tissue weakness – hernia, scoliosis
Propensity to vascular thrombosis
Progressive mental retardation (70%)

Diagnosis is by plasma and urinary amino acids.

Treatment aims to reduce the homocystine levels. Options include pyridoxine, folic acid, a low protein diet and aspirin as an anti-thrombolytic.

Marfan's syndrome

The incidence of Marfan's syndrome is between 1:16,000 and 1:60,000. Inheritance is autosomal dominant, with the gene locus on chromosome 15.

Clinical features of Marfan's syndrome

Usually abnormal at birth
Long fingers, lower segment of the body longer than the upper segment, arm span greater than height
Subluxed lens – upwards and outwards, myopia, retinal detachment, glaucoma and cataract
Hyperextendable joints
Connective tissue weakness – hernia and scoliosis
Mitral and aortic valve disease including aortic root dilatation
Pneumothorax

Diagnosis is clinical. Slit lamp examination and echocardiography are useful. Plasma amino acids exclude homocystinuria.

Cardiac problems are a significant cause of morbidity.

Ectopia lentis
This is an isolated finding of a dislocated lens usually inherited as an autosomal dominant condition.

82. CONGENITAL HYPOTHYROIDISM Answer: CD

This has an incidence of 1 in 4000. It is usually asymptomatic until 6–12 weeks of age. The male to female ratio is 1:2. Symptoms and signs include poor feeding, constipation, lethargy, jaundice, large tongue, umbilical hernia and hoarse cry. Without treatment myxoedema (soft tissue accumulation) and failure to thrive will occur and cretinoid facies will develop.

Neonatal screening is with the Guthrie card test for phenylketonuria at 7–10 days. In most areas both T4 and TSH are assayed. Usually T4 will be low and TSH raised although in 10% the T4 will be normal. Neonatal screening will not usually detect hypothyroidism due to TSH deficiency.

Congenital hypothyroidism is usually due to thyroid dysgenesis sometimes with ectopic thyroid tissue being present. Less commonly it occurs secondary to an inborn error of hormone synthesis (dyshormonogenesis).

Treatment is lifelong with thyroxine. The dose is 100 μg/m^2/day. The best monitoring is growth and development. A normal T4 should be aimed for, but the TSH does not necessarily have to be normal. A high TSH and a normal T4 suggest poor compliance.

Outcome is near normal (but not normal) development provided treatment is started early. Large cohort studies show a 5–10 point difference in IQ compared with a control population. The TSH at presentation is of prognostic importance with the higher levels being of greater concern.

83. KLINEFELTER'S SYNDROME Answer: BD

This has an incidence of 1 in 1000 males. The karyotype is 47 XXY. The aetiology is meiotic non-disjunction with the extra X chromosome coming from the father in 50% and the mother in the other 50%. Increased maternal age is a risk factor. There are a number of variants with more than two X chromosomes and mosaicism is common.

Children are usually asymptomatic until the age of 5 years. After that they can present with behavioural problems or psychiatric disturbance. Intelligence is below average. The children are usually tall and thin. Puberty is delayed and infertility is very common and is due to azospermia. The testes and phallus are small. Gynaecomastia is common (80%). There is an increased risk of pulmonary disease, varicose veins, breast cancer, leukaemia and mediastinal germ cell tumours.

The prepubertal hormone profile is normal. By mid-puberty the FSH and LH are raised and the testosterone is low and testosterone replacement is required. Elevated levels of oestradiol with a high oestradiol: testosterone ratio account for the development of gynaecomastia during puberty.

84. TURNER'S SYNDROME   Answer: ACE

The incidence is 1 in 1500–2500 live born females. Chromosomes 45XO, 45XO/46XX. Mosaicism is present within most cell lines. Paternal sex chromosome is lost. Loss of the maternal sex chromosome is a lethal deletion. No effect of increasing maternal age on incidence.

Spontaneous fetal loss is very common usually in the first trimester.

Clinical features of Turner's syndrome
Infants are usually small for dates
Lymphoedema and feeding difficulties in the neonatal period
Neck webbing
Cubitus valgus
Cardiac abnormalities – coarctation of the aorta, bicuspid aortic valve, aortic stenosis
Renal abnormalities – pelvic kidney, single kidney, pelvic-ureteric junction obstruction
Growth failure
Failure of puberty (hypergonadotrophic hypogonadism)
Pigmented naevi

There are two options for management of growth failure:

- Steroid treatment – oxandrolone, an anabolic steroid with minimal androgenic side effects, if used in low dose will increase final adult height.
- Growth hormone – recombinant growth hormone is given as injections and increases final height (6–8 cm). Higher doses are needed than in growth hormone deficiency.

Management of pubertal failure

20% of Turner's have some ovarian function and develop some signs of puberty. Most require oestrogen replacement at 12–13 years. Once puberty is initiated, cyclical therapy with oestrogen and progesterone leads to menstrual cycles. Successful pregnancies have been described with ovum induction and *in vitro* fertilisation.

85. PHENYLKETONURIA   Answer: ACDE

The metabolic block is the conversion of phenylalanine to tyrosine due to a deficiency of phenylalanine hydroxylase. Incidence is around 1 in 5000. Inheritance is autosomal recessive and carrier detection and prenatal diagnosis are possible.

Infants are normal at birth. Clinical features in the untreated patient are:

- Low IQ
- Poor head growth
- Seizures
- Fair skin 'dilute pigmentation' – due to inadequate melanisation
- Eczema-like rash

Diagnosis is by measuring the plasma phenylalanine which will be raised. The urine has a mousy, pungent odour due to the presence of phenyl acetic acid which is a metabolite of phenylalanine.

Screening is carried out on all babies born in the UK by the Guthrie card which is used to collect a drop of blood which is then used to measure the whole blood phenylalanine by a bacterial inhibition assay. This is done at 4–5 days, ideally after a feed.

Treatment is with a diet that is selectively low in phenylalanine. The diet needs to be lifelong, particularly during pregnancy when untreated or partially treated phenylketonuria is teratogenic to the unborn child. The teratogenicity manifests as severe mental retardation with microcephaly.

86. BONE AGE   Answer: BDE

The bone age defines skeletal maturation and if compared with chronological age gives an idea of growth potential. A child with a delayed bone age compared with chronological age has more growth potential than a child whose bone age equals the chronological age. The bone age, chronological age and height can be used to predict final adult height using special tables (e.g. Bayley-Pinneau).

An X-ray of the left wrist is used to assess bone age. There are two systems in use:
*   Greulich and Pyle system – comparing epiphyseal centres of the left hand and wrist to those in a text book. The knee is sometimes used in younger children.
*   TW2 system – where each epiphyseal centre is scored and the sum of the scores gives an estimate of the bone age.

Causes of delayed bone age
Constitutional short stature
Growth hormone deficiency
Androgen deficiency
Cortisol excess
Turner's syndrome
Chronic disease e.g. asthma, cystic fibrosis, chronic inflammatory bowel disease, coeliac disease
Malnutrition

Causes of advanced bone age
Hyperthyroidism
Androgen excess
   Congenital adrenal hyperplasia
   Precocious puberty
Oestrogen excess
Cerebral gigantism – Sotos syndrome

Familial short stature is a common cause of short stature in children. Parents' heights are usually on the lower centiles. Growth velocity is normal and bone age equal to chronological age.

Constitutional growth delay is slow growth with delayed puberty. Height velocity is normal but height, pubertal development and bone age are 2–4 years delayed. A family history is common and catch up does occur.

Growth hormone excess has no effect on bone age, but causes an increase in linear growth.

87. NOONAN'S SYNDROME   Answer: ABD

This has an incidence of 1 in 1000–2,500 live births. It occurs in both males and females. It is usually sporadic but occasionally familial (autosomal dominant with variable expressivity). The gene defect has been isolated on chromosome 12.

Clinical features of Noonan's syndrome
Normal at birth
Neonatal feeding difficulties
Short stature and delayed puberty
Cardiac defects (pulmonary stenosis, peripheral pulmonary artery stenosis, PDA, ASD)
Broad or webbed neck
Chest defect deformity (pectus carinatum or pectus excavatum)
Cubitus valgus
Characteristic facies (hypertelorism, anti-mongoloid slant, micrognathia, high arched palate, ptosis)

The majority of females are fertile. Direct transmission from parent to child occurs in 30–70%. In males, cryptorchidism is often present which may lead to inadequate secondary sexual development.

Bleeding problems occur in 20%. Mild to moderate mental retardation occurs in 30%.

88. GYNAECOMASTIA   Answer: ABE

Breast tissue grows whenever the ratio of oestrogens to androgens is increased relative to normal adult values. This occurs in most newborn males due to maternal hormones. It also occurs in some males in early puberty when there is an increase in circulating oestrogen which occurs before the surge in masculinising hormones occurs.

Differential diagnosis
Physiological pubertal gynaecomastia
Familial gynaecomastia
Klinefelter's syndrome
Hypergonadotrophic hypogonadism

Hepatic tumours and cirrhosis
Thyroid disease
Starvation
Adrenal/testicular tumours

Drugs
    Steroids
    Tricyclics
    Cimetidine
    Spironolactone
    Cytotoxics
    Exogenous oestrogens

89. PRADER-WILLI SYNDROME   Answer: BC

The incidence is 1 in 10 000. Occurrence is sporadic and associated with a deletion in the long arm of chromosome 15.

The condition goes through three main phases; an initial infantile hypotonic phase, followed by a childhood obese phase and then an adolescent phase during which behavioural problems predominate.

Clinical features of Prader-Willi syndrome
Reduced fetal movements/infantile hypotonia
Dysmorphic features
Childhood hyperphagia and obesity
Short stature, delayed bone age, hypogonadism and infertility
Low IQ
Diabetes mellitus

Life expectancy is reduced as a consequence of the obesity and associated cardiac and respiratory complications.

90. CONGENITAL ADRENAL HYPERPLASIA   Answer: ACDE

The incidence is 1 in 5000. Inheritance is autosomal recessive. The gene defect is known and is part of the HLA complex on chromosome 6. Antenatal diagnosis is possible by either chorionic villous sampling or by amniocentesis.

95% of defects are due to 21 hydroxylase deficiency, 75% of which are salt losers. 11 beta hydroxylase deficiency is the second commonest type and associated with hypertension after the first few years.

Presentation can be in any of the following ways:
- salt losing crises
- premature isosexual development (boys – small testes, large penis and scrotum)
- virilisation in females
- hypertension (11 beta hydroxylase deficiency)

Characteristic features of a salt losing crisis include a low plasma sodium and chloride and a raised potassium with an elevated plasma renin and low plasma aldosterone.

Diagnosis is by:
- Raised plasma 17 hydroxy progesterone and raised urinary pregnantriol (21 hydroxylase deficiency)
- Raised plasma 11-deoxycortisol and 11-deoxycorticosterone (11 beta hydroxylase deficiency).

Treatment is by steroid replacement therapy. Hydrocortisone to replace corticosteroid activity. Fludrocortisone to replace mineralocorticoid activity.

Monitoring of treatment is controversial and includes:
- Measurement of growth
- Bone age
- Blood pressure
- Plasma electrolytes
- Steroid biochemistry (plasma 17 OH progesterone profiles in 21 hydroxylase deficiency)

91. GROWTH HORMONE DEFICIENCY   Answer: AD

The incidence of growth hormone deficiency is 1 in 4000. The male to female ratio is 2:1. The majority of cases are idiopathic.

Aetiologies of growth hormone deficiency
Genetic – primary defect in growth hormone production
Congenital abnormality – associated with midline defects e.g. septo-optic dysplasia, cleft lip and palate
Acquired – perinatal/postnatal infections, CNS infection, radiotherapy
Neoplasia – craniopharyngioma, glioma

Trauma – perinatal, basal skull fracture
Autoimmune

Treatment of growth hormone deficiency is with growth hormone replacement therapy by injection. Growth hormone will increase the final adult height in children with proven growth hormone deficiency. It also increases the final adult height in Turner's syndrome and probably in children with renal failure. Growth hormone therapy has also been given for short stature due to emotional deprivation, skeletal dysplasia and familial short stature although the results have been disappointing with no improvement in final adult height.

92. GROWTH HORMONE   Answer: ABE

Pharmacological stimuli of growth hormone secretion
Insulin
Arginine
Glucagon
L Dopa
Clonidine
Prostaglandin E2
Bombesin
Galanin
GHRH
Strenuous exercise

Provocation tests of growth hormone secretion are potentially hazardous. Insulin tolerance tests are now only performed in specialist centres because of the risk of severe hypoglycaemia. Other stimuli of growth hormone secretion such as glucagon and clonidine have important side effects, glucagon causes vomiting and general fatigue and late hypoglycaemia, clonidine causes drowsiness and hypotension.

93. PRECOCIOUS PUBERTY   Answer: BCD

The commonest forms of sexual precocity are early breast development (thelarche) or the appearance of pubic or axillary hair (adrenarche).

Isosexual (appropriate for sex) precocious puberty can be either true (central, gonadotrophin dependent) or false (gonadotrophin independent).

True precocious puberty is 10 times more common in girls than in boys. It is said to have occurred if the changes of puberty occur before the age of 8 years in girls and 9 years in boys.

Central (true) precocious puberty
This is gonadotrophin dependent and occurs as a consequence of the premature activation of gonadotrophin pulsatility which causes the onset of puberty. It is characterised by accelerated growth, advanced bone age and pubertal levels of LH, FSH and the sex steroids oestrogen and testosterone. It is usually idiopathic in girls (80%), an underlying aetiology being much more common in boys. A CT head scan is indicated in all boys.

Aetiologies
Idiopathic
Hamartoma
Neurofibroma
Glioma
Hydrocephalus
Post trauma
Post meningitis/encephalitis
Prolonged untreated hypothyroidism

False or gonadotrophin independent precocious puberty is characterised by a lack of consistency between different aspects of pubertal development, for example pubic hair and acne with no testicular development. Examples include congenital adrenal hyperplasia, oestrogen producing ovarian tumour, adrenal tumour and medication including anabolic steroids and the oral contraceptive pill.

94. FRAGILE X SYNDROME   Answer: ABD

Fragile X syndrome is a common disorder among mentally handicapped individuals (6% males, 0.3% females). The fragile site is on the long arm of chromosome X at Xq27.3. Inheritance is X linked, but expression is due to the process of allelic expansion. The fragile X locus normally has 2800 trinucleotide base repeats, a small increase in the repeats makes it unstable and through successive generations there is an expansion in the repeats (female transmission increases the repeats) until the increase becomes clinically significant resulting in the fragile X syndrome.

Clinical features include: mental retardation (IQ 30–55 in males, mild mental retardation in females), prominent jaw, long face, large ears, macro-orchidism, hypotonia and joint laxity. The testicular enlargement is more prominent post puberty. Psychological features include cluttering of speech, hyperactivity, emotional instability and autistic features.

Other disorders associated with allelic expansion include
- Huntingdon's disease (male transmission increases the repeat)
- myotonic dystrophy (maternal transmission increases the repeat)

In both disorders an increase in the repeat increases the severity of the disease with onset at an earlier age.

95. GALACTOSAEMIA   Answer: BCDE

Galactosaemia is a rare autosomal recessive disorder. The incidence is around 1 in 50 000 live births.

Three separate defects have been described:
- Galactokinase deficiency which causes cataracts only
- Galactose-1-phosphate-uridyltransferase deficiency. Mild – Duarte variant in which there are no symptoms, but erythrocyte galactose-1-phosphate-uridyltransferase activity is reduced
- Severe galactose-1-phosphate uridyltransferase deficiency – widespread, generalised disorder which produces mental retardation, failure to thrive, cataracts, jaundice, hypoglycaemia and hepatomegaly. There is a rapid progression to irreversible severe mental retardation and cirrhosis in undiagnosed patients.

Severe galactose-1-phosphate-uridyltransferase is the most common presentation. It usually presents in the neonatal period. Reducing substances are present in the urine after the first feed. This is detectable on testing with clinitest tablets. Urine dipstick for glucose is negative.

Diagnosis is confirmed by measuring the enzymes. Treatment is with a lactose free diet. Outcome is variable. Some degree of mental retardation is usual. A number are severely retarded.

96. ALDOSTERONE   Answer: A

Aldosterone is produced in the zona glomerulosa of the adrenal cortex. Secretion is regulated by activation of the renin-angiotensin system. Renin production occurs in the juxtaglomerular apparatus in response to a drop in serum sodium or a fall in blood pressure.

The effect of aldosterone is on the sodium-potassium exchange pump in the distal tubules of the kidney. It acts to increase absorption of sodium from the distal tubule in exchange for potassium or hydrogen ions. Increased sodium absorption increases water absorption and increases blood pressure.

Hypoaldosteronism results in a low serum sodium and a high serum potassium with a low aldosterone and high renin. Deficiency of aldosterone occurs in adrenal hypoplasia, inborn errors of steroidogenesis, Addison's disease, adrenoleukodystrophy, exogenous steroid withdrawal, destruction of adrenal gland (e.g. haemorrhage, tuberculosis) or drugs which cause increased steroid metabolism (e.g. rifampicin, ketoconazole, phenytoin, phenobarbitone).

Pseudohypoaldosteronism is due to end organ resistance to aldosterone. It results in hyponatraemia, hyperkalaemia with a raised renin and aldosterone.

97. NORMAL PHYSIOLOGICAL AND ENDOCRINE CHANGES OF PUBERTY   Answer: AD

In the three years prior to puberty low levels of pulsatile LH become detectable during sleep. LH and FSH are produced in the anterior pituitary and released due to pulsatile gonadotrophin releasing hormone (GnRH) secreted by the hypothalamus. There is an increase in the amplitude and frequency of LH secretion as puberty approaches which causes enlargement of the gonads.

In males, the testicles produce testosterone and in girls the ovaries produce oestradiol and ovarian androgens which with the adrenal androgens produce secondary sexual characteristics.

Onset of puberty is 11 years in girls. The first sign is breast bud development, followed by the appearance of pubic hair 6–12 months later. Menarche usually occurs 2 to 2.5 years after breast bud development. Peak height velocity in girls occurs at breast stage 2–3 and virtually always precedes menarche.

Onset of puberty in boys is 11.5 years. The first sign is testicular enlargement (greater than 3 ml) and thinning of the scrotum. This is followed by pigmentation of the scrotum and growth of the penis. Pubic hair follows. Peak height velocity (growth spurt) is two years later in boys than in girls and occurs at testicular stage 4–5, which is around 13–14 years of age. Breast enlargement occurs in 40–60% of boys (significant enough to cause social embarrassment in 10%) and is a result of oestradiol produced by the metabolism of testosterone. It usually resolves within 3 years.

During puberty, elongation of the eye often occurs causing short sightedness.

98. INSULIN DEPENDENT DIABETES (TYPE ONE)   **Answer: E**

Insulin dependent diabetes mellitus (type one diabetes) occurs as the result of destruction of pancreatic islet cells. Clinical symptoms occur when there is approximately 20% of islet cell activity remaining.

Pathogenesis is thought to be autoimmune. 80–90% of newly diagnosed diabetics have islet cell antibodies. There is an association with HLA antigens: HLA-B8, HLA-BW15, HLA-DR3 and HLA-DR4 (each of these give a 2–3 fold increased risk of developing insulin dependent diabetes). Homozygosity to the absence of aspartic acid in the HLA-DQ beta chain confers a 100-fold increased risk.

Siblings of an affected individual are at a 1–7% risk of developing insulin dependent diabetes (annual UK incidence 7.7 per 100 000). There is a seasonal variation in incidence with peaks during the autumn and winter months. There is also an increased incidence after Coxsackie, mumps and rubella epidemics suggesting that an initial viral infection triggers an autoimmune response against islet cells. There is a peak incidence at age 5–7 years (when children start school and exposure to viral infection increases) and at puberty.

Treatment with immunosuppressive agents has been found to lengthen the honeymoon period. The risks of treatment are greater than the benefits of starting insulin later.

99. COMPLICATIONS OF INSULIN DEPENDENT   **Answer: BCDE**
DIABETES MELLITUS

Complications can be acute or chronic, acute complications being hypoglycaemia, hyperglycaemia and ketoacidosis. Complications can be grouped according to systems:
- CNS – diabetic coma, hypoglycaemia, mood change and irritability

- Peripheral nervous system – mononeuropathies (facial nerve the most common), peripheral neuropathy, sensory loss
- Musculoskeletal – proximal myopathy, joint contractures
- Vascular – peripheral vascular disease, ischaemic heart disease, hypertension
- Eyes – cataracts, retinopathy, acute myopia with hyperglycaemia which recovers with treatment
- Renal – urinary tract infection, nephropathy
- Skin – lipohypertrophy, lipoatrophy, skin infections, vaginal candidiasis
- Autoimmune – thyroid disease, Addison's disease, coeliac disease
- Growth – pubertal delay (with poor control), excess weight gain (with poor dietary compliance), weight loss (due to poor control or inadequate intake), short stature, Mauriac syndrome
- Pregnancy – increased risk of intrauterine death, congenital anomalies, macrosomia and neonatal hypoglycaemia

Mauriac syndrome
This is insulin dependent diabetes associated with dwarfism. The dwarfism is associated with a glycogen-laden enlarged liver, osteopenia, limited joint mobility, growth failure and delayed puberty. It is due to under insulinisation.

100. GRAVES' DISEASE   **Answer: BCD**

Graves' disease is thyrotoxicosis associated with eye manifestations. 5% of cases present in childhood, the peak incidence being during adolescence. There is a female predominance (5:1). A family history is common. There is an association with HLA B8, HLA DR3.

Clinical features of Graves' disease
Emotional disturbance
Irritability
Poor attention span
Tremor
Tachycardia
Increased appetite
Weight loss
Diarrhoea
Goitre
Exophthalmus and ophthalmoplegia
Lid lag
Cardiac involvement (rare in childhood)

T3 and T4 are elevated, TSH is low. TSH receptor stimulating antibodies are usually present at diagnosis and disappear as the condition remits.

Approximately half of childhood cases will remit spontaneously within 2–4 years. Many will progress to become clinically hypothyroid. Medical treatment is with carbimazole and propranolol (the latter to control acute symptoms). Block replacement means that both carbimazole and thyroxine are used. Definitive treatment (favoured by many) is either by subtotal thyroidectomy or the use of radioactive iodine. Severe eye disease may require treatment with prednisolone.

Neonatal thyrotoxicosis is a transient condition resulting from the placental transfer of thyroid stimulating antibodies from a thyrotoxic mother.

Other diseases associated with HLA B8/DR3
Addison's disease
Insulin dependent diabetes mellitus
Coeliac disease
Chronic active hepatitis
Systemic lupus erythematosus
Dermatomyositis
Autoimmune thyroiditis
Primary sclerosing cholangitis

101. HYPERKALAEMIA   Answer: BC

The following are useful in the emergency treatment of acute hyperkalaemia.
- Intravenous calcium gluconate which antagonises the effects of potassium on the heart by stabilising the myocardium. It does not lower the serum potassium. It should be used if either an arrhythmia or the ECG changes of hyperkalaemia are present. Dose 0.1 mmol/kg i.v.
- Salbutamol either intravenously or nebulised. Nebulised dose 2.5 – 10 mg, i.v. dose 4 µg/kg. Salbutamol results in potassium entry into the cell.
- Intravenous sodium bicarbonate. Dose 2.5 mmol/kg i.v. Give if pH <7.3. Sodium bicarbonate promotes the uptake of potassium into cells. In addition, acidosis will impair myocardial function and needs to be corrected. Need to check calcium as if patient is hypocalcaemic, bicarbonate may lower the ionised calcium, precipitating tetany, convulsions, hypotension or arrhythmias.
- Glucose insulin infusion. Dose dextrose 0.5 g/kg/hr and insulin 0.05 u/kg/hr i.v. Promotes the uptake of potassium into cells.
- Ion exchange resin – such as calcium resonium which facilitates sodium potassium exchange in the gut and can be given orally or by enema. Dose 1g/kg initially and then 1g/kg/day.
- Dialysis/haemofiltration.

Hydrocortisone is not useful.
Adenosine is used to control supra-ventricular tachycardia.

ECG changes of hyperkalaemia
Prolongation of the PR interval
Peaked T waves
Widening of the QRS complex
ST depression
Ventricular fibrillation

102. NOCTURNAL ENURESIS   Answer: BC

Nocturnal enuresis is defined as bed wetting for three or more nights per month or one night per week.
- At age 5–6 the prevalence is 8–10%
- At age 7–10 years the prevalence is 5–7%

The male to female ratio is 2:1. After age 10 the male to female ratio gradually disappears. 20–30% are secondary (i.e. start after a period of full night time control for 6 months). The incidence doubles when the father or mother has had nocturnal enuresis and if both parents suffered there is a 70% chance that the offspring will be affected.

Treatment of nocturnal enuresis
General
    Explanation and reassurance
    Diary of wetting
Specific
    Under age 5 years
        Reassurance that all is normal
        Family therapy
        Practical help
    5–7 years
        Star chart
        Lifting
        Desmospray/desmotabs
    Over 7 years
        Star chart
        Desmospray/desmotabs
        Enuresis alarm

Over 7 years of age about 60% using alarm will achieve dryness within 2 months.

DDAVP (desmopressin) as either spray or tablets has a success rate of 60–70% but a high relapse rate when the treatment is stopped (30%). In children under 7 years of age DDAVP may relieve stress in the family in the short or long term. An adequate fluid intake must be maintained when on DDAVP and the medication should be stopped if vomiting occurs in order to prevent severe hyponatraemia. Desmospray 20–40 µg at bed time. Desmotabs 0.2–0.4 mg at night.

103. BERGER'S DISEASE   Answer: ACE

Berger's disease is part of the differential diagnosis of recurrent haematuria. It is a histological diagnosis. The diagnosis is made when the predominant feature on renal biopsy is granular deposition of IgA and C3 in the mesangium of the glomerulus in the absence of systemic disease e.g. systemic lupus erythematosus or abnormal plasma immunoglobulins or complement levels. The male to female ratio is 2:1.

It usually presents with haematuria following an upper respiratory tract infection. Microscopic haematuria may persist. Macroscopic haematuria is associated with upper respiratory tract infections. Proteinuria occurs in 40–50%.

The prognosis for most children is good. 5–10% will develop end stage renal failure. Poor prognostic features include heavy proteinuria, hypertension and proliferative lesions on renal biopsy.

Deafness is not a feature. Deafness is a feature of Alport's syndrome.

Berger's disease commonly recurs in transplanted kidneys.

104. RENAL FAILURE   Answer: B

In pre-renal failure there is a reduction in the intravascular volume which results in a reduced glomerular filtration rate. This activates the renin-angiotensin system and results in the secretion of aldosterone which promotes sodium reabsorption and potassium excretion in the distal tubule.

Intravascular depletion results in a more concentrated urine being passed. This urine is characterised by a high osmolality (greater than 500 mosm/l) and a low sodium (less than 20 mmol/l). The urine plasma: creatinine ratio is high (greater then 40).

The fractional excretion of sodium is calculated as follows:

$$\frac{\text{Urine Na x Plasma Cr}}{\text{Urine Cr x Plasma Na}} \times 100 \ (\%)$$

Urine Na = urinary sodium
Urine Cr = urinary creatinine
Plasma Na = plasma sodium
Plasma Cr = plasma creatinine

The fractional excretion of sodium is less than 1% in pre-renal failure and greater than 1% in renal failure.

In neonates, sodium reabsorption is less efficient and the fractional excretion of sodium is nearer to less than 2.5% in pre-renal failure and greater than 2.5% in renal failure.

This approach is not helpful if either mannitol or diuretics have been given which will interfere with the urinary electrolytes.

Diarrhoea can precede pre-renal (e.g. gastroenteritis) failure or renal (haemolytic uraemic syndrome) failure.

105. RENAL OSTEODYSTROPHY   Answer: AB

Renal osteodystrophy is a potentially life-threatening complication of chronic renal failure. A reduction in glomerular filtration rate causes a reduction in the excretion of inorganic phosphate. The decline in renal function reduces the production of 1,25 dihydroxy vitamin D from 25 hydroxy vitamin D decreasing calcium absorption from the gut. Hyperphosphataemia and low serum calcium stimulate parathyroid hormone secretion (secondary hyperparathyroidism). Parathyroid hormone
- Increases calcium reabsorption in the distal tubule
- Decreases phosphate reabsorption in the proximal tubule
- Stimulates the synthesis of 1,25 dihydroxy vitamin D in the proximal tubule
- Promotes osteoclastic bone reabsorption.

The biochemical features of renal osteodystrophy
Normal or low serum calcium
Increased plasma phosphate
Increased plasma alkaline phosphatase
Markedly increased parathyroid hormone level
Normal or reduced 25 hydroxy vitamin D
Reduced 1,25 dihydroxy vitamin D

The management is dietary phosphate restriction, use of a phosphate binder (such as calcium carbonate, aluminium hydroxide) and 1 alpha hydroxy cholecalciferol or 1, 25 dihydroxycholecalciferol.

Vitamin D
Sources are diet and ultraviolet radiation. Vitamin D is hydroxylated to 25 hydroxy vitamin D in the liver. 25 hydroxy vitamin D is further hydroxylated to 1,25 dihydroxy vitamin D in the kidney. 1,25 dihydroxy vitamin D promotes:
- Calcium resorption from bone
- Calcium and phosphate reabsorption from the kidney
- Calcium and phosphate absorption from the gut
- Cell growth and differentiation.

	Vitamin D deficiency	Hypophosphataemic rickets	Renal osteodystrophy
Calcium	reduced	normal	normal
Phosphate	reduced or normal	reduced	increased
Alkaline phosphatase	increased	increased	increased
PTH	increased	normal	markedly increased

106. HENOCH-SCHOENLEIN PURPURA　　　　　Answer: A

20–50% of children with Henoch-Schoenlein purpura have renal involvement. This is usually mild with microscopic haematuria and proteinuria although a nephrotic or a nephritic picture may occur in up to 2%. The renal manifestations are usually present within the first month but can present later and almost always present within 3 months. Careful follow-up of blood pressure, urine microscopy and plasma creatinine is required in patients with renal involvement until the manifestations of this disappear.

Renal biopsy should be considered if
• There is significant and persistent proteinuria
• The patient develops frank nephrotic syndrome
• There is evidence of renal insufficiency
High dose immunosuppression is given to those with severe renal involvement.

There is no diagnostic test for Henoch-Schoenlein purpura. The differential diagnosis includes
• Systemic lupus erythematosus
• Post streptococcal glomerulonephritis
• Haemolytic uraemic syndrome

Systemic lupus erythematosus is suggested by the clinical picture, a low C3, C4 and ANA positivity. In children with post streptococcal glomerulonephritis there is usually a history of preceding streptococcal infection. The laboratory features include a low C3 and a raised ASO titre. The blood film in haemolytic uraemic syndrome is characteristic.

The prognosis of Henoch-Schoenlein nephritis depends on the extent of glomerular lesions. Poor prognostic factors include:
- Clinical evidence of renal insufficiency
- Clinical evidence of nephrotic syndrome
- Glomerular sclerosis
- Glomerular necrosis
- Extensive crescent formation

107. SYNDROMES   Answer: B

Nephrogenic diabetes insipidus
This is an X linked recessive condition characterised by resistance of the kidney to the anti-diuretic action of anti-diuretic hormone. The symptoms and signs include polyuria, polydipsia, dehydration, failure to thrive and mental retardation. The plasma biochemistry is characteristic and shows hypernatraemia, hyperchloraemia and hyperosmolality. Diagnosis is by a water deprivation test which demonstrates a failure to concentrate the urine despite exogenous anti-diuretic hormone. Treatment includes a low salt diet, hydrochlorothiazide and indomethacin.

Alport's syndrome
Alport's syndrome is inherited as an X linked dominant with occasional families showing an autosomal dominant inheritance pattern. It is characterised by haematuria, progressive impairment of renal function, deafness, ocular manifestations and a characteristic appearance on renal biopsy. The disease is usually silent in childhood and presents in adolescence with microscopic haematuria and proteinuria. Males are more severely affected than females.

Hartnup disease
This condition has an autosomal recessive inheritance pattern. It is characterised by a tubular and intestinal defect in the reabsorption and absorption of cyclic and neutral amino acids. The clinical features of the condition are secondary to tryptophan malabsorption. These include a photosensitive rash and cerebella ataxia. The condition is diagnosed by the demonstration of a specific pattern of amino aciduria. Tryptophan malabsorption results in a nicotinamide deficiency and treatment with nicotinamide corrects the clinical features.

Vitamin D resistant rickets
This is an X linked dominant condition which usually present between 12 and 18 months. The plasma biochemistry demonstrates a normal

plasma calcium, low phosphate, raised alkaline phosphatase, normal parathyroid hormone level and vitamin D level. Treatment is with phosphate and vitamin D.

Cystinosis
This is an autosomally recessively inherited condition. It can present in the infant, adolescent or adult. The presentation in infancy is with failure to thrive, recurrent vomiting and dehydration. The biochemistry is of a metabolic acidosis with a low plasma potassium and a low plasma phosphate. The diagnosis is made by measurement of the white cell cystine. Treatment is with potassium and bicarbonate replacement as with other Fanconi type syndromes and additionally with phospho-cysteamine. It is important to differentiate cystinosis from cystinuria. Cystinuria is an inborn error of the metabolism of dibasic amino acids. Low cysteine solubility leads to renal stone formation. This is the only complication. The stones are radio-opaque.

108. NEPHROTIC SYNDROME   Answer: C

Minimal change nephrotic syndrome
This has a male predominance. It is rare in the first year of life. Peak incidence is in the age range 2–5 years. It can occur in adult life. Haematuria is usually absent. The presence of haematuria implies that a more serious form of glomerulonephritis should be considered as does the presence of hypertension or abnormal renal function tests. Complement levels are normal.

Complications of nephrotic syndrome
Hypovolaemia
Hypertension
Infection
Thrombosis
Hyperlipidaemia
Acute renal failure

Referral to a paediatric nephrologist should be considered if
Age less than 12 months
Age greater than 10 years
Macroscopic or persistent microscopic haematuria
Impaired renal function not attributable to hypovolaemia
Hypertension

Differential diagnosis of nephrotic syndrome in children aged 1–15 years
Minimal change nephrotic syndrome
Focal segmental glomerulosclerosis
Mesangiocapillary glomerulonephritis
Membranous nephropathy
Henoch-Schoenlein nephritis
Systemic lupus erythematosus

109. METABOLIC ACIDOSIS   Answer: DE

Pyloric stenosis
Hypochloraemic metabolic alkalosis.

Cystinuria
Defect in the intestinal absorption and renal tubular reabsorption of the dibasic amino acids cystine, lysine, arginine and ornithine. The consequence is the formation of renal calculi. Treatment is to alkalinise the urine.

Bartter's syndrome
The basic defect of Bartter's syndrome is impaired tubular chloride reabsorption. The biochemical features are of hypokalaemia, hypochloraemia, alkalosis, hyperreninaemia and hyperaldosteronism associated with a normal blood pressure and high urinary losses of potassium and chloride.

Cystinosis
This condition is discussed elsewhere, the biochemical features being metabolic acidosis associated with a high plasma chloride and a low potassium and phosphate.

Pseudohypoaldosteronism
Pseudohypoaldosteronism is characterised by unresponsiveness of the distal tubule to aldosterone. Hyponatraemia, hyperkalaemia and dehydration occur. Metabolic acidosis can occur (type IV renal tubular acidosis).

110. URINARY TRACT INFECTION   Answer: ABE

Urinary tract infection in childhood always requires investigation. There is no consensus plan for this and that listed below represents just one approach.

Plan of investigation

Under 2 years	USS, DMSA, MCUG
2–5 years	USS, DMSA
Over 5 years	USS

Further investigation is indicated in children over the age of 2 years if
- USS abnormal
- Recurrent infections
- Acute pyelonephritis
- Family history of reflux

A Mag III indirect cystogram can be used to look for vesico-ureteric reflux and for renal scars once continence has been achieved. A DMSA scan is a static scan which will detect renal scars. A DTPA is a dynamic scan. The indication for it is to look for obstruction at any level of the renal tract and uses frusemide to promote a diuresis.

Prophylactic agents
Trimethoprim 2 mg/kg at night
Nitrofurantoin 1 mg/kg at night

111. HAEMOLYTIC URAEMIC SYNDROME   Answer: CDE

Haemolytic uraemic syndrome is on the increase. Peak age is 1–2 years. Peak incidence occurs during the summer months. 50% require dialysis in the acute phase and mortality is of the order of 5–10%. Hyponatraemia occurs in 70% and thrombocytopenia in 50%. The blood film shows a microangiopathic haemolytic anaemia.

There are two subgroups within the syndrome:

D+ (95%)
Prodromal diarrhoea
Associated with verotoxin producing *E. coli* 0157:H7.
Other associated infections include Coxsackie virus, *Shigella* dysentry, streptococcal infection.
85% make a full recovery
Neutrophilia (>15) predicts a difficult course

D– (5%)
Often familial
No prodromal illness
Runs relapsing course
70% progress to chronic renal failure

112. RENAL TUBULAR ACIDOSIS   Answer: ADE

Proximal renal tubular acidosis

This occurs as a result of a failure of reabsorption of bicarbonate in the proximal tubule. It is characterised by a high urinary pH, low plasma bicarbonate and metabolic acidosis. Most patients with proximal renal tubular acidosis manifest this tubular abnormality as part of the Fanconi syndrome. In patients with proximal renal tubular acidosis distal tubular acidification is intact. This means that following an acid load the urinary pH will drop below 5.5.

Fanconi's syndrome

This is a generalised transport abnormality in the proximal tubule characterised by excessive urinary losses of amino acids, glucose, bicarbonate, phosphate, calcium, magnesium and uric acid. It is characterised by metabolic acidosis, dehydration, hypokalaemia, hypophosphataemia, rickets and growth retardation. There are many causes both hereditary and acquired.

Treatment

The treatment of proximal renal tubular acidosis is large amounts of alkali as sodium bicarbonate and sodium citrate. The Fanconi syndrome requires treatment as appropriate with phosphate, potassium and vitamin D.

Distal renal tubular acidosis

This occurs as a consequence of reduced hydrogen ion secretion in the distal tubule. It is not possible to lower the urinary pH below 5.5 regardless of the acid load. Children present with unexplained acidosis, failure to thrive, nephrocalcinosis, rickets and polyuria. Hypokalaemia and hypercalciuria are both common and can be severe. The treatment is with sodium and potassium bicarbonate. The condition can be autosomal dominant, sporadic or secondary.

113. PROTEINURIA
Answer: ABC

Orthostatic
Increased protein in the urine in the upright posture, absent when lying flat. Proteinuria is variable but can be large. It is a benign condition. Renal function is normal and family history negative.

Intermittent
Intermittent proteinuria is common after exercise or stress and with no obvious precipitant. It is rarely of serious significance.

114. HAEMATURIA
Answer: ACD

There are many causes of haematuria. The haematuria itself can be macroscopic, intermittent or microscopic. Haematuria needs to be distinguished from other conditions like excessive beetroot ingestion, rifampicin, haemoglobinuria and myoglobulinuria which produce red urine.

Causes of haematuria
Infection
Trauma
Glomerulonephritis
Hypercalciuria
Renal calculi
Hydronephrosis and other congenital abnormalities
Vascular problems
Tumours
Bleeding disorder
Drug induced e.g. cyclophosphamide
Exercise induced
Factitious

The coexistence of proteinuria with haematuria makes a renal parenchymal lesion more likely. Heavy proteinuria suggests glomerular disease. Ultrasound and plain abdominal radiography are essential to exclude obstruction, calculi or tumours. A family history of deafness suggests Alport's syndrome.

115. HYPERTENSION
Answer: ABE

To measure the blood pressure manually the blood pressure cuff should cover half of the upper arm. A small cuff will result in a high reading.

Causes of hypertension in childhood
Acute glomerulonephritis
Chronic glomerulonephritis
Reflux nephropathy
Haemolytic uraemic syndrome
Polycystic renal disease
Coarctation of the aorta
Renal artery stenosis
Phaeochromocytoma
Congenital adrenal hyperplasia/11 beta hydroxylase deficiency
Acute hypovolaemia
Essential hypertension

Drug treatment of hypertension
Diuretics e.g. frusemide
Calcium channel blockers e.g. nifedipine
Angiotensin converting enzyme inhibitors e.g. captopril
Vasodilators e.g. prazosin, hydralazine, sodium nitroprusside
Beta blockers e.g. propranolol
Alpha and beta blockers e.g. labetalol

Complications of hypertension
Left ventricular failure
Retinopathy
Hypertensive encephalopathy

Emergency treatment of hypertensive encephalopathy
Nifedipine
Labetalol IV
Sodium nitroprusside

116. ACUTE POST-STREPTOCOCCAL GLOMERULONEPHRITIS

Answer: AC

This commonly follows group A beta-haemolytic streptococcal infection. The ASOT (anti-streptolysin titre) is positive in 90% which is indicative of recent streptococcal infection. The ASOT may not rise after a skin infection whereas anti-DNAse B will rise irrespective of infection site. There are other implicated infectious agents which are less commonly seen.

The usual age of presentation is between 2 and 10 years; it is commoner in males. The classical presentation is of preceding upper respiratory tract infection followed by the onset of macroscopic haematuria and oedema after 2 weeks indicating an acute nephritis. Oliguria is usually present for the first 10 days of the nephritic illness.

The C3 is low initially and returns to normal within 6–12 weeks. C4 is less frequently low and if so returns to normal much quicker.

Problems include hypertension, pulmonary oedema and renal insufficiency. Treatment is with oral penicillin for 10 days to eradicate the streptococcus. This does not influence the time course or severity of the nephritis. Diuretics may be required. Steroids are not indicated.

Feature of acute nephritis
Haematuria
Proteinuria
Oedema, ascites, pleural effusions
Hypertension
Renal insufficiency

Differential diagnosis of acute nephritis in childhood
Post-infectious glomerulonephritis
Henoch-Schoenlein nephritis
IgA nephropathy
Alport's syndrome
Lupus nephritis

117. UNDESCENDED TESTIS   Answer: ADE

The testis are undescended in 3% of babies born at term and 1% at the age of 12 months. Spontaneous descent is very rare after the first birthday. True undescended testis must be distinguished from retractile testis which can be 'milked' down into the scrotum. Impalpable testis are not necessarily absent and may be intra-abdominal. The incidence of undescended testis is much higher in preterm babies. 30% of cases are bilateral.

There is an increased risk of infertility and of malignancy in children with undescended testis. In order to minimise these, orchidopexy should be carried out before the end of the second year. The incidence of testicular tumours in adults is 3 per 10,000. The risk in males with a history of undescended testis is 4–40 times greater. 60% of the tumours are seminomas, most of the remainder being teratomas.

Important associations of undescended testis include:
Spinal muscular atrophy
Myotonic dystrophy
X linked icthyosis
Kallmann's syndrome
Prune belly syndrome

118. WILMS' TUMOUR   Answer: BCE

There is an increased risk of Wilms' tumour in the following conditions:
- Isolated hemihypertrophy
- Beckwith Wiedemann syndrome
- Neurofibromatosis
- Drash syndrome
- WAGR syndrome
- Sporadic aniridia
- Aniridia associated with deletion of the short arm of chromosome 11

Drash syndrome
Ambiguous genitalia
Nephropathy
Wilms' tumour, often bilateral

WAGR syndrome
Wilms' tumour
Aniridia
Genitourinary malformations
Mental retardation

Wilms' tumour accounts for 10% of all paediatric tumours and 22% of abdominal masses in childhood. 10% are bilateral. Ultrasound is the best investigation to make the diagnosis. The prognosis is good, with 80–90% 5 year survival.

119. CHLORIDE   Answer: CDE

Chloride is the major anion of extracellular fluid. The reabsorption of tubular fluid must be isoelectric. Sodium and potassium transfer with chloride and bicarbonate. Chloride is actively transported in the ascending limb of the loop of Henlé and in the gut. Chloride and bicarbonate act such that if extracellular chloride is reduced then bicarbonate reabsorption is increased (hypochloraemic metabolic alkalosis) and if bicarbonate is reduced in the extracellular fluid chloride reabsorption is increased (hyperchloraemic metabolic acidosis).

Hypochloraemia (<95mmol/l)
Loss of hydrochloric acid from the stomach results in a metabolic alkalosis and volume depletion. This activates the renin-angiotensin system and promotes sodium reabsorption (with bicarbonate as chloride is depleted) in the proximal tubule and sodium exchange for potassium and hydrogen ions in the distal tubule.

Hyperchloraemia
Three settings:
- Excessive intake
- Increased absorption from the gastrointestinal tract
- Renal tubular acidosis

Excessive chloride in the extracellular fluid will suppress bicarbonate reabsorption and lead to the development of a metabolic acidosis. Renal tubular acidosis manifest by a bicarbonate leak will increase chloride reabsorption.

120. HYPONATRAEMIA   Answer: CDE

Antidiuretic hormone (ADH) is synthesised by the hypothalamus and released from the posterior pituitary gland. Synthesis is stimulated by an increase in the extracellular osmolality. The hormone itself enhances water reabsorption from the collecting tubules and so dilutes the extracellular osmolality.

Diabetes insipidus occurs when there is a failure of ADH either to be produced (cranial diabetes insipidus) or to act (nephrogenic diabetes insipidus). This leads to hypernatraemia with an inappropriately dilute urine. Common symptoms are polyuria and polydipsia. Cranial diabetes insipidus can be either idiopathic or secondary to damage to the hypo-thalamopituitary axis secondary to either a head injury or a tumour. Nephrogenic diabetes insipidus can be either congenital (usually X linked) or acquired (secondary to intoxications or systemic disease). Its pathogenesis is a failure of ADH to act on the collecting tubules. A water deprivation test is required to differentiate cranial diabetes insipidus, nephrogenic diabetes insipidus and psychogenic polydipsia. In the latter a dilute urine is produced as a consequence of excess drinking. If following water deprivation the urine is concentrated then the diagnosis is psychogenic polydipsia, if not and the urine concentrates in response to exogenous ADH then the diagnosis is cranial diabetes insipidus. If the urine fails to concentrate in response to either manoeuvre then the likely diagnosis is nephrogenic diabetes insipidus.

There are many causes of inappropriate ADH secretion which include severe infection, serious illness, post surgery and CNS disorders. The condition presents with fluid retention and oliguria. Hyponatraemia occurs and the serum is hypo-osmolar. The diagnosis is made by the finding of an inappropriately high urine osmolality with a low serum osmolality. Treatment is with fluid restriction.

Plasma osmolality = 2 x (plasma sodium + plasma glucose + plasma urea)

Causes of hyponatraemia
Inappropriate i.v. fluids
Excessive loss in the urine, faeces, vomit or sweat
Prematurity
Inadequate intake
Inappropriate ADH secretion
Salt losing state e.g. congenital adrenal hyperplasia, Addison's disease
Renal tubular acidosis
Diuretic therapy

121. MEMBRANEOUS GLOMERULONEPHRITIS   Answer: ACE

Males predominate in this condition which represents under 1% of childhood nephrotic syndrome but 20–40% of adult nephrotic syndrome. It can present with full blown nephrotic syndrome or with mild proteinuria and haematuria.

It can be idiopathic or secondary to other diseases such as systemic lupus erythematosus or hepatitis B. The C3 is initially low in membranous glomerulonephritis due to either of these conditions.

Steroids are beneficial in the adult but rarely so in childhood. Progression to renal failure is very rare.

Causes of secondary membranous nephropathy
Hepatitis B
Malaria
Schistosomiasis

Leprosy
Systemic lupus erythematosus
Mercury
Gold
Sickle cell disease
Rheumatoid arthritis

Other types of glomerulonephritis which present as nephrotic syndrome
Focal segmental glomerulosclerosis
Mesangiocapillary (membranoproliferative) glomerulonephritis
Mesangial proliferative glomerulonephritis

122. POLYCYSTIC KIDNEY DISEASE   Answer: BCE

Autosomal recessive polycystic renal disease usually presents in the first year of life. The incidence is 1 in 40 000. The commonest presentation is with either respiratory distress or enlarged kidneys in the neonatal period. Ultrasound is the best method of diagnosis. Death often occurs rapidly although a number survive and those that do so beyond the first year generally do well.

Autosomal dominant polycystic renal disease accounts for 8% of adults in end-stage renal failure. The incidence is between 1 in 200 and 1 in 1000. The gene is on chromosome 16. It usually present in adult life but can, rarely present in the neonatal period. The renal cysts are associated with cysts in other organs including the liver, pancreas spleen and lungs. 10% have a beri aneurysm in the circle of Willis.

123. VESICO-URETERIC REFLUX   Answer: BCD

30–40% of children who present to hospital with a confirmed urinary tract infection have vesico-ureteric reflux (boys > girls). Of those, up to 30% develop renal scars. The diagnosis is by micturating cystography. Severity is graded from I to IV, with grade IV implying intra-renal reflux is present. A Mag 111 indirect cystogram can be used once continence has been achieved but this is both less sensitive and less specific although a better tolerated procedure.

The object of management is to prevent urinary tract infections and in doing so prevent renal scarring (reflux nephropathy). This is best achieved using low dose prophylactic antibiotics to prevent infections and appropriate antibiotics if breakthrough infection occurs based on urine culture and sensitivity.

Most reflux resolves by the age of 5 years. If not and recurrent infections occur with progressive renal scarring then ureteric re-implantation is indicated. DMSA is the best investigation to look for renal scars.

Complications of reflux nephropathy
Hypertension
Left ventricular failure
Impaired renal function
Renal failure

124. HYPERCALCIURIA   Answer: ABD

Hypercalciuria is important as it is a risk factor for the production of renal calculi and can cause other urinary symptoms including polyuria, nocturnal enuresis and dysuria. It is also commonly associated with microscopic haematuria.

The gold standard is to measure the 24 hour urinary calcium (upper limit of normal 0.1 mmol/kg/day); the measurement of the urinary calcium creatinine ratio is also useful (upper limit of normal 0.7).

Causes of hypercalciuria
Normocalcaemic
Hypercalcaemic

Normocalcaemic
Idiopathic (familial)
Distal renal tubular acidosis
Frusemide

Hypercalcaemic
Increased bone resorption
    Immobilisation
    Steroids
    Primary hyperparathyroidism
    Thyroid disease
    Cushing's disease

Increased intestinal absorption
   Calcium
   Vitamin D
Hypophosphataemia
William's syndrome

William's syndrome
Typical elfin facies
Failure to thrive
Supravalvular aortic stenosis, peripheral pulmonary stenosis
Hypercalcaemia, hypercalciuria
Familial or sporadic, usually the latter
Mild intellectual impairment

125. CONGENITAL NEPHROTIC SYNDROME   Answer: AE

The commonest congenital nephrotic syndrome is the Finnish type. Incidence is 12 per 100,000 live births. Babies are often born preterm, small for gestational age and have a large placenta. Proteinuria often occurs *in utero* and the alphafetoprotein is raised. 30% develop oedema in the first week of life with abdominal distension and ascites.

Renal function is normal initially but deteriorates to end-stage renal failure within the first 2 years of life. Renal biopsy is characteristic. There is no available treatment. Patients are managed with regular albumin transfusions followed by bilateral nephrectomy, dialysis, high calorie feeding and renal transplantation.

126. IRON DEFICIENCY ANAEMIA   Answer: B

The commonest cause of iron deficiency anaemia in childhood is dietary. Iron is absorbed in the proximal small intestine. It is usually the case that about 10% of the ingested load is absorbed. This can be increased by the simultaneous administration of vitamin C. Iron deficiency anaemia is particularly common in the first year of life. Both breast and cows' milk are low in iron and iron-rich foods such as fortified cereals and infant formula milks need to be taken.

The symptoms and signs of iron deficiency include pallor, fatigue, pica and poor appetite, the latter exacerbating the problem. Splenomegaly is present in 10–15%. There is much recent evidence which suggests that iron deficiency even in the absence of anaemia is a cause of reduced intellectual performance and that this responds well to therapy.

Laboratory features
Microcytosis
Hypochromia
Low serum iron
Increased total iron binding capacity
Low serum ferritin
Thrombocytosis (occasional thrombocytopenia)

Treatment is with oral iron. A reticulocyte response should be seen within a few days. 6 mg/kg/day of elemental iron is required. Chronic blood loss needs to be considered as an alternative cause of iron deficient anaemia particularly if stools are positive to blood or there are suggestive features in the history. Beta thalassaemia trait is an important differential diagnosis.

Beta thalassaemia trait
HbA2 3.4–7%   Normal adult 1.5–3.5%
HbF 2–6%   Normal adult < 2%
HbA2 levels are low in iron deficiency anaemia.

Iron absorption
Iron is absorbed in its ferrous form (approximately 10% of intake) according to body needs. This process is aided by gastric juice and vitamin C and inhibited by fibre and steatorrhoea. Iron is transported in plasma in the ferric state bound to transferrin. It is stored in liver, spleen

bone marrow and kidney as ferritin. Following breakdown of haemo-globin the iron is conserved and reused.

127. ACUTE IDIOPATHIC THROMBOCYTOPENIC PURPURA
Answer: E

Incidence is 4 per 100 000 children per year. Peak age is 2–4 years. Incidence in boys and girls is equal. Commonest in the winter and spring, and often preceeded by an upper respiratory tract infection. It is probably immune mediated although the precise mechanism is not known.

Differential diagnosis
Infection
Drugs
Collagen disorders
Familial thrombocytopenia
Leukaemia
Aplastic anaemia
Portal hypertension with hypersplenism

Investigations are determined by the clinical history and physical examination. A full blood count and blood film is essential in all cases. Other investigations are as appropriate. A bone marrow is required if there is doubt about the diagnosis and leukaemic infiltration is a possibility or if steroids are going to be used. This in particular is a subject of much debate at the moment.

Bed rest is not helpful. Treatment options include steroids, intravenous immunoglobulin (IVIG) or nothing. Steroids and IVIG will increase the platelet count in about 12 hours. Currently IVIG is the preferred option the dosage is variable but generally either 0.8 g/kg as a one off dose, 400 mg/kg for 5 days or 1 g/kg for 2 days.

Chronic idiopathic thrombocytopenia occurs more commonly in girls and is defined as the persistence of the thrombocytopenia beyond 6 months. Treatment options include steroids, regular IVIG and splenec-tomy.

Intracranial haemorrhage is a rare complication of idiopathic thrombo-cytopenic purpura.

128. GLANZMANN'S THROMBASTHENIA
Answer: BC

This is autosomally recessively inherited, with the gene locus on chromosome 7. Pathogenesis is a failure of platelet aggregation in response to ADP, collagen and thrombin. This is due to a defect in glycoprotein IIb and IIIa both being part of the platelet membrane and deficiency resulting in a failure of the platelet to bind fibrinogen.

It is a very rare condition and presents in early childhood with recurrent bleeding. Platelet count and platelet morphology is normal. The only possible long term treatment is bone marrow transplantation. In the short term tranexamic acid can be used to control acute bleeding.

Bernard Soulier syndrome
This is an autosomal recessive condition. The characteristic features are giant platelets with a reduced life span and hence thrombocytopenia and a prolonged bleeding time. Platelet aggregation is normal.

129. HEREDITARY SPHEROCYTOSIS
Answer: AC

The incidence is 1 in 5000 people of Northern European extraction. It is inherited as an autosomal dominant with variable penetrence. It usually presents in childhood with the classical triad of anaemia, jaundice and splenomegaly. The jaundice is unconjugated and worsens with viral infections. Pigmented gallstones are present in 85% by the second decade. Neonatal jaundice is common. Aplastic crises can occur.

The diagnosis is made on clinical grounds, by observing the spheroidal cells on a blood film and by the increased osmotic fragility of red cells when tested.

Treatment is symptomatic or by splenectomy. The spleen is the site of red cell destruction. Removal of it will reduce haemolysis and reduce the incidence of gallstones. There is however an increased risk of pneumococcal and other infection with splenectomy and pneumococcal vaccine and lifelong prophylactic penicillin needs to be given.

Glucose 6 phosphate dehydrogenase deficiency
X linked inheritance. Can either present with an acute haemolytic crises or as a chronic haemolytic anaemia. Neonatal jaundice is common. Diagnosis is by estimation of the glucose 6 phosphate dehydrogenase level (can be normal during a crisis). Management is by avoidance of precipitating factors. Infection may also provoke a crisis.

Substances to avoid
Fava beans
Antimalarials
Sulphonamides
Dapsone
Nitrofurantoin
Nalidixic acid
Methylene blue
Naphthalene

130. WISKOTT ALDRICH SYNDROME

Answer: CDE

This has an X linked inheritance. The gene has been localised to the short arm of the X chromosome. Prenatal diagnosis and carrier detection is possible in 98%.

Clinical features of Wiskott Aldrich syndrome
Recurrent infections secondary to immunodeficiency
Eczema
Thrombocytopenia with reduced platelet size
Malignant potential

Laboratory investigations
Reduced platelet number and reduced platelet size
Low serum IgM, normal Ig G and raised IgA and IgE
T cell defect

Acute haemorrhage is a significant cause of death (20%), other causes being infection and malignancy. Survival beyond the teenage years is rare. Bone marrow transplant is the only possible cure.

TAR syndrome
Autosomal recessive
Absent radii
Thrombocytopenia
Variable other manifestations including cardiac, renal, gastrointestinal, and skeletal.

131. VITAMIN B12 DEFICIENCY

Answer: A

To be absorbed vitamin B12 must combine with intrinsic factor which is secreted by the parietal cells of the stomach. The complex is then absorbed in the terminal ileum.

Symptoms and signs of B12 deficiency
Megaloblastic anaemia
Smooth tongue
Ataxia
Hyporeflexia
Up going plantars

Pernicious anaemia is the commonest cause of B12 deficiency in adults. It is due to deficiency of intrinsic factor and is associated with either parietal cell or intrinsic factor antibodies. These are not detected in children with juvenile pernicious anaemia.

The Schilling test is used to assess the absorption of vitamin B12 from the gut.

Other causes of B12 deficiency
Nutritional e.g. vegans
Infants of vegan mothers particularly if breast fed
Inflammatory bowel disease
Tuberculosis affecting the terminal ileum
Surgical resection of the terminal ileum e.g. necrotising enterocolitis
Bacterial overgrowth (blind loop syndrome)

The mean corpuscular volume is raised in vitamin B12 deficiency.
B12 deficiency is rare in coeliac disease at presentation.

132. SICKLE CELL DISEASE   Answer: ABCDE

Sickle cell disease is due to synthesis of an abnormal haemoglobin. There are various forms, Hb SS is the most common and the most severe. Sickling occurs during hypoxia which causes the abnormal haemoglobin to crystallise making the red cell stiff. This then blocks the microcirculation causing infarction.

Clinical expression is varied, some patients leading an almost normal life. *In utero* diagnosis can be made by chorionic villus sampling at 10 weeks. Diagnosis at birth can be made on heel prick or cord blood. This allows early follow-up and treatment.

Crises due to sickling are precipitated by anoxia, cold, infection and dehydration. Painful vascular occlusive crises occur in bone, the common sites being hips, shoulders, vertebrae and the bones of the hands and feet. Sickling can also result in pulmonary infarction, splenic infarction (causing hyposplenism), gut infarction and cerebrovascular accidents. Treatment of a crisis involves intravenous antibiotics, intravenous fluid, oxygen, analgesia and sometimes blood transfusion. Acute sequestration of blood may occur in the spleen or lung (acute chest syndrome) causing an acute anaemia. An aplastic crisis can occur secondary to infection with parvovirus B19.

Functional hyposplenism occurs. Prophylactic penicillin and pneumococcal immunisation (after the third birthday) need to be given. Although often large in the first few years the spleen reduces in size throughout childhood as a consequence of autoinfarction.

Nocturnal enuresis is common (45% of 8 year olds). Growth rate is reduced but puberty delayed resulting in a reasonable final height in most cases.

Mortality is low in the first 6 months, peaks between 6–12 months and falls after first year. In Jamaica mortality is 5% by first year, 25% by 20 years. The commonest cause of death is infection.

133. RHESUS HAEMOLYTIC DISEASE   Answer: CDE

Haemolytic disease of the newborn occurs as a consequence of the transplacental passage of anti-D antibodies (IgG) from the rhesus negative mother to the rhesus positive fetus. This can only occur if the mother has been sensitised. Other rhesus antibodies (e.g. anti C and E) can occur and produce less severe disease.

The use of anti-D passive immunisation in mothers within 72 hours of delivery has reduced the incidence of the disease. Sensitisation in the mother (rhesus negative) can occur following miscarriages, abortions and previous deliveries of rhesus positive fetuses.

Haemolytic disease can occur *in utero* and may produce hepatosplenomegaly, ascites and hydrops (which can be detected on ultrasound). Screening is done on rhesus positive mothers at booking, 28, 34 weeks and at time of delivery. If anti-D antibodies are found the tests are repeated every 2 weeks. If titres are high (greater than 10 iu/ml) referral to a specialist centre is indicated. Titres above 100 iu/ml indicate severe disease.

If the anti-D antibody titres are high then *in utero* monitoring of the fetus is carried out by amniocentesis to measure bilirubin levels in the amniotic fluid. If amniotic bilirubin levels indicate a high degree of haemolysis is present (plotted on a Liley chart) then cord blood sampling is performed. Fetal anaemia will be the consequence of severe haemolysis and can be treated with *in utero* blood transfusions. Severe disease is an indication for premature delivery (at 34–36 weeks), the infant being likely to require exchange transfusion after birth.

The severity of disease will increase with successive pregnancies.

ABO haemolytic disease

This usually occurs in mothers with blood group O who have IgG anti-A or anti-B antibodies which will cross the placenta and react if the baby is blood group A or B and cause haemolysis. The degree of haemolysis is generally only mild. It occurs in 3% of births. Phototherapy usually controls the jaundice. Diagnosis is by measuring anti-A or anti-B antibodies in a blood group O mother with a blood group A, B or AB neonate with a positive direct Coombs' test.

134. ANAEMIA SECONDARY TO CHRONIC DISEASE   Answer: CD

Anaemia can occur in any disease with chronic inflammation. Characteristic features include:
- Normal MCV
- Normochromia
- Normal or low reticulocyte count
- Low serum iron
- Low iron binding capacity and transferrin saturation
- Normal or raised ferritin
- Increased reticuloendothelial stores of iron

Several factors are thought to contribute to the anaemia including decreased red cell survival, inflammatory mediators suppressing erythrocyte production, a blunting of the erythropoietin response to anaemia and trapping of iron by macrophages reducing utilisation for new red cells. Anaemia is usually not less than 9 g/dl.

Although most cases will not respond to iron, supplements are given if serum ferritin is less than 50 µg/ml and may improve anaemia if there is coexistent iron deficiency.

Anaemia secondary to chronic renal failure is due to absence of erythropoietin production and responds to treatment with recombinant erythropoietin.

135. NEONATAL THROMBOCYTOPENIA   Answer: ACDE

Causes of neonatal thrombocytopenia
Congenital
    TAR (thrombocytopenia, absent radii) syndrome
    Fanconi's anaemia
    Bernard Soulier syndrome
    Wiskott-Aldrich syndrome
Immune mediated platelet destruction
    Maternal ITP
    Neonatal isoimmune thrombocytopenia
    Maternal systemic lupus erythematosus
Due to congenital infection
    TORCH
    Congenital syphilis
Sepsis
Polycythaemia
Drugs e.g. Tolazoline

Neonatal isoimmune thrombocytopenia
This occurs in neonates who are platelet antigen (PL A1) positive born to PL A1 negative mothers. Sensitisation occurs *in utero* and first pregnancies can be affected. 2% of the population are PL A1 negative, 98% are PL A1 positive but only 6% of PL A1 negative mothers with positive fetuses will develop antibodies. 10% of affected fetuses will have intraventricular haemorrhage with a high associated morbidity and mortality. Monitoring of maternal antibodies can be performed during pregnancy and platelet transfusion of PL A1 negative platelets given to infants at risk.

136. TRANSFUSION REACTIONS   Answer: BCDE

Transfusion reactions can be immediate or delayed.

Immediate reactions
Haemolysis
Reaction to infected blood
Allergic reactions to platelets or white cells (causing urticaria)

Pyrogenic reactions to plasma proteins or transfused antibodies
Clotting abnormalities after large transfusions
Circulatory overload
Citrate toxicity
Hyperkalaemia

Late reactions
Transmission of infection e.g. hepatitis A, B and C, HIV, cytomegalo-
virus, brucella, salmonella, toxoplasma, malaria.
Iron overload
Immune sensitisation

Reactions can be mild with pyrexia normally due to reactions to white
cells, platelets or transfused plasma proteins and usually occurring in
patients receiving multiple transfusions. Treatment is with i.v. hydrocortisone and antihistamines. If the reaction is more severe the
transfusion should be stopped. Adrenaline may occasionally be required.
Transfusion reactions can be reduced by using white cell depleted blood
or using white cell filters. Clinical features of severe reactions include
abdominal pain, back pain, flushing, headache, shortness of breath,
pyrexia, rigors, chest pain, vomiting and shock.

137. NEUTROPENIA   Answer: ABDE

Neutropenia is classified as either <1.0 x10^9/l or <0.5 x10^9/l neutrophils.

Causes of neutropenia
Congenital
    Reticular dysgenesis – failure of development of stem cells
    X linked hypogammaglobulinaemia – neutropenia in a third of cases
    Kostmann's syndrome – severe neutropenia (<0.2 x10^9/l
    Schwachmann's syndrome
    Cartilage-hair hypoplasia
    Fanconi's anaemia
Neutropenia associated with metabolic disorders
    Propionic acidaemia
    Isovaleric acidaemia
    Methylmalonic acidaemia
    Hyperglycinaemia

Immune mediated
  Neonatal isoimmune
  Autoimmune neutropenia e.g. systemic lupus erythematosus
  Drugs
Others
  Infection
  Drugs - chemotherapy
  Felty's syndrome (neutropenia, leukopenia, rheumatoid arthritis and
  splenomegaly)
  Cyclical neutropenia

Chronic granulomatous disease
Chronic granulomatous disease is a defect of neutrophils which are
unable to kill ingested bacteria. The condition is very rare (incidence 1
in a million). Inheritance is autosomal recessive in 35% and X linked in
65%. Diagnosis is by the failure of neutrophils to change the yellow dye
NBT (nitro blue tetrazolium) blue.

Fanconi's anaemia
Autosomal recessive disorder presenting between 3–10 years of age with
thrombocytopenia and variable pancytopenia. There are many associated
features which include abnormal pigmentation, short stature, renal
anomalies and mental retardation. There is an increased risk of leukaemia.

138. CAUSES OF BONE PAIN AND ANAEMIA   Answer: ABCDE

Vitamin C deficiency (scurvy)
The majority of cases occur between 6 and 24 months of age. Deficiency
results in impairment of the formation of collagen. Symptoms are of
irritability, loss of appetite, tachypnoea and generalised bone tenderness
due to sub-periosteal haemorrhages. Haemorrhage may also occur in the
skin, bone, subdural space and gut. Other features include poor wound
healing, bluish purple spongy swelling of the gums and haematuria. X-
ray changes may be seen in the long bones around the knee with white
lines seen on the ends of the shafts of the femur and tibia. Areas of bone
destruction may also be seen.

Neuroblastoma
Accounts for 8% of childhood cancer. Incidence 1 per 100,000. Median
age at onset is 20 months. The tumour arises from primitive neural crest
cells and can arise anywhere in the sympathetic nervous system. The
commonest site is the adrenal medulla. Other sites include the cervical

and thoracic sympathetic chains. Metastases can occur anywhere with bone pain, cord compression, mediastinal mass, metastases to skin, liver and bone marrow with bone marrow suppression and pancytopenia. Production of catecholamines may produce hypertension and products detected on urine testing include vanillymandelic acid (VMA) and homovanillic acid (HVA). Prognosis is dependent upon staging, and the age at presentation.

Langerhans cell histiocytosis

Langerhans cell histiocytosis is the previously described histiocytosis X which encompasses Letterer-Siwe disease, Hand-Schuller-Christian disease and eosinophilic granuloma. Syndromes are identified according to the degree or number of organ systems involved for example Langerhans cell histiocytosis, solitary skull lesion instead of eosinophilic granuloma. Children presenting with generalised Langerhans cell histiocytosis can have involvement of many organ systems.

139. ACUTE LYMPHOBLASTIC LEUKAEMIA Answer: ABCE

Acute lymphoblastic leukaemia (ALL) accounts for one-third of childhood malignancies in the UK. The overall risk of ALL is 1 in 3500 in the first 10 years of life. There is a peak incidence between 2–6 years of age with boys affected more than girls (ratio 1.2:1.0).

There seems to be a genetic factor. In affected individuals the risk of an identical twin developing ALL is 14–20%, the risk of a sibling developing ALL is 1 in 900.

Clinical symptoms at presentation include fever (60%), lethargy, bone pain, bruising, abdominal pain, anorexia and CNS involvement (2.5%). Signs include pallor and bruising, lymphadenopathy and hepatosplenomegaly. An anterior mediastinal mass is present in 5–10%.

Investigations include anaemia (70%), thrombocytopenia (70%), neutropenia in nearly all patients and a high white count (>50 x10^9/l in 20%). Chest X-ray may show mediastinal mass, pleural effusions or cardiomegaly. CSF examination shows leukaemic cells in 5% and implies CNS involvement. The white count at diagnosis is the most important prognostic indicator, with white count >50 x 10^9/l indicating a worse prognosis. Other poor prognostic features include age less than 2 years at diagnosis, CNS involvement, presence of a mediastinal mass and being a boy. Long term survival is around 50%.

140. THROMBOCYTOSIS   Answer: BCE

Thrombocytosis may be:

Physiological (premature infants)
Primary
    Down's syndrome (transient)
    Myeloproliferative disorders
Secondary
    Infection
    Malignancy
    Post-splenectomy (absent splenic pooling)
    Chronic inflammatory disease (juvenile chronic arthritis, ulcerative colitis, Crohn's disease)
    Kawasaki's disease, platelet count raised in 2nd–3rd week of illness
    Iron deficiency
    Vitamin E deficiency
    Rebound thrombocytosis after thrombocytopenia (e.g. due to disseminated intravascular coagulation, chemotherapy).

141. APLASTIC ANAEMIA   Answer: ABCDE

Aplastic anaemia is pancytopenia resulting from aplasia of the bone marrow with no evidence of extramedullary disease.

Causes of aplastic anaemia
Congenital
    Schwachmann syndrome
    Dyskeratosis congenita
Acquired
    Idiopathic (majority)
    Drugs (chloramphenicol, sulphonamides, gold, cytotoxics)
    Ionising radiation, chemicals and toxins (e.g. benzene, organic solvents, insecticides)
    Viral infections (e.g. hepatitis A and C, parvovirus, HIV, Epstein-Barr virus)
    Pre-leukaemic states
    Pregnancy

Aquired aplastic anaemia has an incidence of 1 per million with a male to female ratio of 2:1. Onset is often acute and prognosis can be poor.

142. DISEASES WITH AN INCREASED RISK OF MALIGNANCY
Answer: ABCDE

Ataxia telangiectasia – leukaemia or lymphoma in 10%
Bloom syndrome – risk of leukaemia or other malignancy in 25%
Down's syndrome – risk of leukaemia in 1 in 74
Fanconi's anaemia – leukaemia in 1 in 12
Hemihypertrophy and Beckwith-Wiedemann syndrome – adrenal carcinoma, Wilms' tumour, hepatoblastoma
Chediak-Higashi syndrome – risk of lymphoma
Gardner syndrome/familial adenomatous polyposis coli – carcinoma of colon
Xeroderma pigmentosum – increased risk of skin cancer
Neurofibromatosis – CNS tumours in 5–10%
Tuberous sclerosis – rhabdomyoma of heart, astrocytomas
Von Hippel-Lindau syndrome – phaeochromocytoma, cerebellar haemangioblastoma and retinal angiomata
Klinefelter's syndrome – breast cancer

143. VON WILLEBRAND'S DISEASE
Answer: ACD

Type I – classical von Willebrand's disease
This has autosomal dominant inheritance; chromosome 12 carries the defect. The pathogenesis is under-production of von Willebrand's protein, the role of which is platelet aggregation and carriage of factor VIII.

Laboratory features include prolonged bleeding time, normal platelet count, normal prothrombin time and prolonged partial thromboplastin time. Diagnostic features include a reduced level of von Willebrand's protein, von Willebrand's activity and factor VIII activity. Platelet adhesion is reduced and platelets do not aggregate when the antibiotic ristocetin is added to platelet rich plasma.

Clinical features reflect the bleeding tendency and include bruising, nose bleeds, bleeding from the gums, menorrhagia and prolonged bleeding after injury. Haemarthrosis is rare but can occur in severe disease. Treatment of bleeding episodes is with fresh frozen plasma or cryoprecipitate; the latter being more effective. DDAVP can be used for mild episodes.

There are other types of von Willebrand's disease (types II and III). These are less common.

Haemophilia
Haemophilia A – factor VIII deficiency (X linked)
Haemophilia B – factor IX deficiency (X linked), Christmas disease
Haemophilia C – factor XI deficiency (autosomal recessive)
Normal platelet function and bleeding time. Normal level of von Wille-brand's factor.

144. BLEEDING TIME   Answer: ADE

The bleeding time assesses platelet function, platelet number and vascular integrity. It is extremely sensitive to platelet number. Normal is between 4 and 8 minutes. The technique is very precise and the common-est cause of a prolonged bleeding time is that this has been done incorrectly, for example too deep a cut has been made or the cuff pressure is too high.

Causes of a prolonged bleeding time
Poor technique
Aspirin
Platelet function disorders
    Glanzmann's thrombasthenia
    Bernard Soulier disease
Thrombocytopenia from any cause
Von Willebrand's disease

If the prolonged bleeding time is not due to a low platelet count then a defect of platelet function should be suspected. Platelet counts of more than $50 \times 10^9/l$ are usually associated with normal bleeding times.

145. X LINKED AGAMMAGLOBULINAEMIA   Answer: ACDE

This is also known as Bruton's disease. It is commoner in males. The gene is localised to the long arm of chromosome X. Prenatal diagnosis is possible. The disorder is characterised by absent or low IgA, G and M. T cell function is normal. It presents after 3–6 months as the fall in transplacentally acquired IgG occurs. Presentation is with recurrent bacterial infection. There is an increased risk of malignancy as with most other immunodeficiencies.

Screening is by doing the serum immunoglobulins in children with recurrent infection. Blood group antibodies and the antibody response to immunisations given will also be absent.

Regular intravenous immunoglobulin is indicated in addition to prompt treatment of infections with appropriate antibiotics. In some patients prophylactic antibiotics are indicated. Bone marrow transplantation is the treatment of choice.

146. DI GEORGE SYNDROME   Answer: BCE

This is usually sporadic although familial clustering has been reported. The gene has been localised to chromosome 22.

Clinical features of Di George syndrome
Thymic aplasia/hypoplasia (hypoplasia is more common than aplasia)
Hypoparathyroidism
    Presents with hypocalcaemic seizures (neonatal tetany)
    Absent PTH
Congenital heart disease
    Right sided aortic arch
    Truncus arteriosus
    Interrupted aortic arch
    Atrioventricular septal defect
    Ventricular septal defect
    Hypoplastic pulmonary artery
    Pulmonary atresia
Facial abnormalities
    Hypertelorism
    Cleft lip or palate
    Low set ears
    Anti-mongoloid slant
Others
    Imperforate anus, oesophageal atresia
    Failure to thrive
    Chronic infection (otitis media, pneumonia, diarrhoea)
    Deafness

The total lymphocyte count can be low, normal or raised. Assessment needs to be made of the percentage of circulating mature lymphocytes by assessing their response to phytohaemoglutinin (PHA).

Treatment first aims to deal with manifestations of the syndrome (hypo-calcaemia, cardiac defects). In the long term, bone marrow trans-plantation is the treatment of choice. Graft versus host disease can occur following cardiac bypass and irradiated blood products need to be given in order to try and avoid this.

147. OSTEOSARCOMA   Answer: C

The male to female ratio is 1.5:1. Peak incidence is in the second decade. There is an increased risk associated with retinoblastoma, previous chemotherapy and radiotherapy. Tumours occur in the metaphyseal region of long bones with the distal femur being the most common site followed by proximal tibia and the proximal humerus. It usually presents with pain. Metastases (lung and bone) are present at presentation in 20%.

Diagnosis is by radiology and biopsy. The bone appearing sclerotic on a plain radiograph. Treatment is with chemotherapy and surgery. Prognosis is 60% cure if metastases are not present at diagnosis and 20% if they are. Differential diagnosis is Ewing's and osteomyelitis.

Ewing's sarcoma
The male to female ratio is 1.5:1. It usually presents in the second decade. There are no known risk factors. Tumours may arise in any bone but are found most often in flat bones (pelvis, chest wall vertebrae) and the diaphyseal region of long bones. The presentation is with local pain and swelling. Fever and a raised ESR are common. The appearance on X-ray is of a lytic lesion affecting the medullary cavity and cortical bone. The tumour elevates the periosteum giving an 'onion skin' appearance. Metastases are present in 25% at presentation. Treatment is with radiotherapy and chemotherapy. Surgery is not always required. Survival depends on whether metastases are present at diagnosis and is 20% cure if they are and 70% if they are not.

Differential diagnosis of a lytic bone lesion
Ewing's sarcoma
Langerhans cell histiocytosis
Osteomyelitis
Lymphoma
Neuroblastoma
Metastatic sarcoma

148. IRON POISONING   Answer: ACDE

Ingestion of 60 mg/kg or more of iron may result in systemic iron toxicity. An abdominal X-ray may be useful to confirm iron ingestion as the tablets are radio-opaque. The effects of iron toxicity are dependent on the time after ingestion:

- Stage one (30 mins–2 hours)
  Local effects of gastrointestinal irritation including diarrhoea and vomiting. Haematemesis and hypotension may occur.
- Stage two (2–6 hours)
  Apparent recovery during which iron absorption and accumulation of iron in tissues and mitochondria occur.
- Stage three (12 hours)
  Cellular and mitochondrial damage occurs with hypoglycaemia and lactic acidosis.
- Stage four (2–4 days)
  Severe hepatic necrosis with raised aspartate aminotransferase, alanine aminotransferase, bilirubin and abnormal prothrombin time.
- Stage five (2–4 weeks)
  Late effects with scarring and stenosis of the pylorus.

Investigation of iron poisoning
Free iron levels in serum
Abdominal X-ray
Although investigations are useful, it is important to consider the child's symptoms as a guide to toxicity.

Treatment
Treatment is general and specific. Emesis and gastric lavage are not useful. Desferrioxamine (iron chelator) is the main therapeutic agent available. Supportive treatment needs to be given for hypotension or shock. If free iron is greater than 50 mg/dl or total iron is greater then 350 mg/dl then parenteral desferrioxamine is indicated. Desferrioxamine can cause anaphylaxis. It causes the urine to turn red while chelated iron is being excreted. Oral desferrioxamine may actually promote iron absorption and should not be used.

149. CARBON MONOXIDE POISONING   Answer: ABD

Carbon monoxide is a tasteless, odourless, colourless and non-irritant gas. It binds to haemoglobin to form carboxyhaemoglobin which reduces the oxygen carrying capacity of the blood and shifts the oxygen dissociation curve to the left. The affinity of haemoglobin for carbon monoxide is 250 times greater than that for oxygen.

Endogenous production occurs and maintains a resting carboxyhaemoglobin level of 1–3%. Smoking increases carboxyhaemoglobin levels. Other sources of raised levels include car exhaust fumes, poorly maintained heating systems and smoke from fires.

Clinical features of carbon monoxide poisoning occur as a result of tissue hypoxia. PaO_2 is normal but the oxygen content of the blood is reduced. Toxicity relates loosely to the maximum carboxyhaemoglobin concentration. Other factors include duration of exposure and age of the patient.

Maximum carboxyhaemoglobin concentration
10%   not normally associated with symptoms
10–30%   headache and dyspnoea
60%   coma, convulsions and death
Neuropsychiatric problems can occur with chronic exposure.

Treatment of carbon monoxide poisoning is with 100% oxygen which will reduce the carboxyhaemoglobin concentration. Hyperbaric oxygen is said to reduce the carboxyhaemoglobin level quicker.

150. TRICYCLIC OVERDOSE   Answer: ACD

The mortality of deliberate tricyclic antidepressant overdose is 7–12%.

Effects of tricyclic antidepressants
Anticholinergic, causing tachycardia, pupil dilatation, dry mucous membranes, urinary retention, hallucinations and flushing.
Adrenergic (early), causing hypertension and tachycardia.
Alpha adrenergic receptor blocking, causing prolonged hypotension.
Central inhibition of neuronal re-uptake of noradrenaline, 5-hydroxy-tryptamine, serotonin and dopamine leading to convulsions and coma.
Cardiac, mainly ventricular tachycardia and fibrillation.
Arrhythmias are the main cause of death.

Treatment of overdose
Initial treatment is aimed at preventing absorption of the drug. Emetics should only be used if there is no CNS depression. Activated charcoal should be given every 2–4 hours.

Arrhythmias may respond to correction of hypoxia and correction of acidosis with sodium bicarbonate aiming for a pH of 7.45–7.55. Anti-arrhythmics are best avoided.

Convulsions should be treated with intravenous diazepam. Diazepam can also be used to treat delirium and agitation during recovery.

Hypotension may respond to treatment with i.v. fluids and colloid.

In overdosage, tissue concentrations quickly rise giving tissue to plasma ratios of between 10:1 and 30:1. The drug in plasma is extensively bound to plasma proteins and removal by dialysis is ineffective.

INFECTIOUS DISEASES AND IMMUNOLOGY
ANSWERS

151. TOXOPLASMOSIS
Answer: BDE

Toxoplasmosis is caused by the protozoan *Toxoplasma gondii*. The primary hosts are members of the cat family. Transmission to man is by ingestion of oocytes from the faeces of infected cats and the consumption of extra-intestinal forms of the parasite from undercooked meats. Toxoplasmosis usually causes a latent infection, recognised on serological testing. Overt infection is rare. Features include:

- Generalised fatigue and myalgia
- Lymphadenopathy (most commonly cervical)
- Arthralgia
- Transient maculopapular rash (rare)
- Hepatosplenomegaly (rare)
- Pneumonia/myocarditis (rare)

More serious manifestations can occur in the immunocompromised host and include ocular manifestation (uveitis, chroidoretinitis), pseudo-tumour cerebri and encephalitis.

Laboratory features include atypical lymphocytosis, inversion of the CD4:CD8 ratio and eosinophilia. Diagnosis is serological, IgM anti-bodies appear within a few days and IgG antibodies within a few weeks. Isolation of *Toxoplasma gondii* from blood, CSF or body secretions is difficult but is also diagnostic.

Treatment, if required, is with a combination of pyrimethamine and sulphadiazine. The former is a folate antagonist and so folinic acid supplementation is required.

Congenital toxoplasmosis

There is a 40% risk of transmission if the mother is infected during pregnancy. The risk of infection is higher the more advanced the pregnancy. However, manifestations are more serious the earlier infection occurs. 90% of congenitally infected infants are asymptomatic in the neonatal period. The classical triad of retinochoroiditis, hydrocephalus and intracerebral calcification is uncommon and the clinical manifestations are usually non-specific. If infection is diagnosed during pregnancy then termination is an option, alternatively spiramycin has been given. Neither pyrimethamine or sulphadiazine can be given during the first trimester of pregnancy as both are teratogenic. They are used later in pregnancy.

152. *STREPTOCOCCUS PNEUMONIAE*   Answer: AC

Pneumococci are Gram-positive diplococci. There are more than 80 distinct serotypes. More than 60% of the population carry pneumo-coccus in their nasopharynx, most of these being strains of low virulence.

Diseases caused by *Streptococcus pneumoniae*
Otitis media
Sinusitis
Scarlet fever
Impetigo
Pneumonia
Septicaemia
Peritonitis
Septic arthritis
Osteomyelitis
Meningitis
Brain abscess

Risk factors for pneumococcal infection
Extremes of age
Sickle cell disease
Immunodeficiency
    Antibody deficiency – hypogammaglobulinaemia, subclass deficiency
    Phagocyte abnormalities – neutropenia, hyposplenism, asplenia
    Complement deficiencies
    HIV
    Leukaemia

Diseases for which the vaccination (Pneumovax) is recommended in children over 2 years
Asplenia, splenic dysfunction, post splenectomy
Sickle cell disease
Diabetes mellitus
Immunodeficiency
Chronic respiratory disease
Congenital heart disease
Chronic renal disease – nephrotic syndrome
Chronic liver disease

There are 23 serotypes which cause 80% of severe infections and it is these that are covered by the pneumococcal vaccine. Protection is not complete. The vaccine lasts for approximately 5 years although the duration of efficacy is not clear.

Antibiotic prophylaxis is indicated in at-risk groups.

Lyme disease is caused by the spirochaete *Borrelia burgdorferi*.

153. ATYPICAL MYCOBACTERIAL INFECTION   Answer: C

Non-tuberculous or atypical mycobacterial infections are seen at the extremes of age. The infective agents are acid fast bacilli found in the environment. Unlike tuberculous infection, atypical mycobacterial infection is acquired from the environment and not from person-to-person contact and hence contact tracing is not helpful.

There are 13 strains of non-tuberculous mycobacteria which can potentially infect man. Common strains include *Mycobacterium avium*, *Mycobacterium intracellulae*, *Mycobacterium marinum*, *Mycobacterium scrofulaceum*. The number of cases per year is increasing possibly due to better case recognition.

Lymphadenitis is the commonest presentation in childhood. This is usually anterior cervical or submandibular. The child usually presents between age 2 and 5 years. The lymphadenopathy is usually unilateral and systemic symptoms are rare. Spontaneous resolution may occur but often not for many months. If the lymphadenitis ruptures then a discharging sinus will develop.

Pulmonary disease is rare in childhood but common in adults. There is an increased incidence in older children with cystic fibrosis. Cutaneous disease is also rare in childhood. The usual agent if it occurs is *Mycobacterium marinum*. Skeletal involvement can occur and usually manifests as infected bursae, tendons and sheaths. Disseminated disease is rare but can occur in children who are immunosuppressed.

Diagnosis requires a high index of clinical suspicion. Intradermal skin tests can be helpful in distinguishing non-tuberculous from tuberculous mycobacterial infection. Incisional biopsy of infected glands is often performed in order to exclude malignancy. However, although reassuring, this often results in sinus formation which can become chronically infected. Excision biopsy is the preferred method of obtaining a histological specimen. Non-caseating granulomas are often seen. Definitive diagnosis is by culture which often takes up to 3 months.

Complete surgical excision is the treatment of choice. If excision is not possible or incomplete then chemotherapy is required. Conventional antituberculous therapy is usually ineffective. First line therapy is with clarithromycin and rifabutin. Second-line therapy includes ethambutol and ciprofloxacin.

Differential diagnosis of cervical lymphadenopathy
Cervical abscess
Tuberculosis
Cat scratch fever
Mumps
Salivary stone
Malignancy
Infectious mononucleosis
Toxoplasmosis
Brucellosis

154. FAMILIAL MEDITERRANEAN FEVER   Answer: BCE

This shows autosomal recessive inheritance with male predominance. The gene is carried on chromosome 16. Onset is usually in the first or second decade. Acute attacks of fever and abdominal pain (peritonitis) are characteristic. Pleuritis and arthritis can occur. 25% suffer skin lesions. The episodes usually occur once or twice a month. Attacks tend to remit during pregnancy but return afterwards.

Colchicine can be used to suppress an attack and should be used at the first sign of prodromal symptoms. Its use as a prophylactic agent can reduce the number of attacks.

Amyloidosis can complicate familial Mediterranean fever and is deposited in the adrenals, spleen, glomeruli, alveoli and in arterioles and veins. The liver and heart are usually spared. Colchicine will reduce the incidence of amyloidosis.

There are no diagnostic tests. The underlying pathology is hyperaemia and non-bacterial inflammation. It is thought to be due to deficiency of a protease which normally inhibits the chemotactic activity of C5a and IL8.

155. VIRUSES   Answer: BC

RNA containing viruses

Arenavirus	Lassa fever
Orthomyxovirus/paramyxovirus	Influenza
	Parainfluenza
	Measles
	Mumps
	Respiratory Syncytial virus
Picornavirus	Enterovirus
	Rhinovirus
Reovirus	Rotavirus
Retrovirus	HIV
Rhabdovirus	Rabies
Rubivirus	Rubella
Togavirus	Hepatitis C
Torovirus	Ebola fever

DNA viruses

Adenovirus	
Hepadnavirus	Hepatitis B
Herpes virus	Cytomegalovirus
	Epstein-Barr virus
	Herpes simplex virus
	Varicella zoster virus
Papovavirus	Papilloma virus
Parvovirus	Parvovirus B19
Pox virus	Molluscum contagiosum

156. CEREBROSPINAL FLUID   Answer: CD

The normal values for CSF cell count, protein, glucose and pressure at different ages should be known and can be found in any standard reference text.

CSF protein is higher in preterm than in term infants and higher in term infants than in children or adults.

Red cells are not a normal finding in the CSF of older children although they may be present as a consequence of the tap being traumatic.

CSF pressure rises with age.

There are many causes of a raised CSF white cell count including tumours. The CSF white cell count and glucose can be normal in bacterial meningitis.

157. IMPETIGO   Answer: ACE

Impetigo can be classified as simple (non-bullous) or bullous. Bullae are usually flaccid, rupture easily and contain pus. The usual infecting agent is *Staphylococcus aureus*. The lesions occur in clusters, are usually found at the extremities and are highly infectious. Non-bullous impetigo is due to either *Staphylococcus aureus* or group A beta haemolytic streptococcus.

Lesions are painless and not usually associated with systemic symptoms. Regional adenitis can occur. Topical antibiotics are not generally helpful and systemic antibiotics are the treatment of choice. Erythromycin or penicillin and flucloxacillin should be used.

158. INFECTIOUS MONONUCLEOSIS   Answer: ABDE

Infectious mononucleosis (glandular fever) is caused by infection with the Epstein-Barr virus. An infectious mononucleosis-like illness can be caused by other agents including cytomegalovirus, adenovirus and toxoplasmosis.

Epstein-Barr infection is often subclinical. Clinical infection is rare in the pre-school group. Spread is by transmission of oral secretions ('kissing disease').

The clinical features are of fever, pharyngitis and lymphadenopathy. The syndrome often persists for some weeks and a post viral fatigue syndrome can occur. The appearance of a maculo-papular rash following the administration of ampicillin is quite characteristic. Splenomegaly is seen in 50%. A smaller number of patients develop mild jaundice and hepatomegaly.

Laboratory features include an atypical lymphocytosis, mild thrombo-cytopenia and a transient elevation of the transaminases. Confirmation is by the Paul Bunnell test or Epstein-Barr virus serology. It is important to realise that (particularly in children under 5 years) the Paul Bunnell test can be negative in glandular fever due to Epstein-Barr virus infection. In such cases the presence of IgM antibody to viral capsid antigen is diagnostic.

Complications are rarely seen but include splenic rupture, airway obstruction, Guillain-Barre syndrome, VII nerve palsy, agranulocytosis and pancarditis. Treatment is supportive.

Infections commonly associated with an atypical lymphocytosis
Cytomegalovirus
Malaria
Toxoplasmosis
Tuberculosis
Mumps

Epstein-Barr virus is associated with
Nasopharyngeal carcinoma
Burkitt's lymphoma
B cell driven lymphomas

159. SCHISTOSOMIASIS   Answer: ABCD

Schistosomes are trematodes that have a mammal as the definitive host and a snail as an intermediate host. The main schistosomes affecting man are *S. haematobium*, *S. japonicum*, *S. mansoni*, *S. intercalatum* and *S. mekongi*. Schistosomiasis is a very common infection worldwide which particularly affects children and young adults in endemic areas. Humans are infected through contact with water contaminated with cercariae, the free-living infective stage of the parasite.

Infection is usually asymptomatic. The manifestations of acute infection are fever, arthralgia, lymphadenopathy, hepatosplenomegaly and a rash. This is immune complex mediated. More serious is chronic infection with retention of eggs in the host and chronic granulomatous injury. The organs affected are the urinary tract and intestine (directly) and liver, lungs and central nervous system by haematogenous spread. Granulomas surround the eggs. Cell mediated responses play a role. Chronic renal failure and bladder carcinoma can result.

S. haematobium usually affects the renal tract and can cause haematuria, frequency and dysuria and obstructive uropathy. *S. japonicum*, *S. mansoni*, *S. intercalatum* and *S. mekongi* usually cause intestinal symptoms, the most common being abdominal pain and bloody diarrhoea. Other manifestations include chronic liver disease and cirrhosis, chronic lung disease and cor pulmonale and spinal cord lesions such as transverse myelitis. Seizures can occur secondary to central nervous system disease.

Diagnosis is by the identification of the eggs in excreta. Eosinophilia is common. Treatment is by eradication of the parasite using Praziquantel.

160. NOTIFIABLE DISEASES

Answer: BCDE

England and Wales 1995
Acute encephalitis
Acute poliomyelitis
Anthrax
Cholera
Diptheria
Dysentery (amoebic or bacillary)
Food poisoning (all sources)
Leprosy
Leptospirosis
Malaria
Measles
Meningitis
Meningococcal septicaemia without meningitis
Mumps
Ophthalmia neonatorum
Paratyphoid
Plague
Rabies
Relapsing fever (*Borrelia* infection)
Rubella
Scarlet fever
Smallpox
Tetanus
Tuberculosis
Typhoid fever
Typhus
Viral haemorrhagic fever
Acute viral hepatitis
Whooping cough
Yellow fever

161. MEASLES

Answer: BCD

Worldwide, measles infection is very common and is associated with significant morbidity and mortality. Measles is caused by an RNA virus. Transmission is person-to-person and by droplet infection. Humans are the only host. It is a notifiable disease. Infection is rare under the age of 6 months due to the presence of maternal antibodies. Second attacks can occur.

Incubation is 14 days from exposure to the appearance of the rash. Infectivity is greatest during the prodromal period and persists for 5 days after the appearance of the rash. The initial symptoms are fever, cough and coryza. The rash is an erythematous maculopapular one. It is widespread and classically starts behind the ears. Koplik's spots in the mouth are pathognomonic. Diagnosis is clinical and by serology.

Complications of measles
Early
    Otitis media
    Laryngotracheobronchitis
    Myocarditis/pericarditis
    Encephalitis
    Primary or secondary (bacterial) pneumonia
Late
    Subacute sclerosing panencephalitis

Prevention of measles is by vaccination. Measles vaccination is given as part of the MMR at around 14 months of age. From October 1996 a pre-school booster has been given because a single dose of vaccine does not confer lifelong immunity.

162. LYME DISEASE   Answer: AC

Lyme disease is a multisystem disease caused by the spirochaete *Borrelia burgdorferi*. Transmission is by infected ticks. Vector hosts include deer and mice. Apart from transplacentally, person-to-person transmission does not occur.

The most common clinical finding is a skin rash (erythema migrans) which begins 4–20 days after the tick bite. Lesions can occur at any site – most cases involve the thigh, buttocks or axilla. Associated with the rash are fever, lymphadenopathy, conjunctivitis, pharyngitis and anicteric hepatitis. Later problems (after weeks or months) include neurological, cardiac and joint involvement. Neurological involvement includes aseptic meningitis, cranial nerve involvement (facial nerve palsy being the most common), peripheral radiculopathy, chorea, cerebella ataxia and Guillain-Barre syndrome. Cardiac involvement is rare, problems seen include atrio-ventricular block, myocarditis and left ventricular dysfunction. Arthritis occurs more commonly. It is usually of sudden onset and can be a mono, oligo or polyarthritis. Arthritis is generally a late manifestation.

The diagnosis is essentially a clinical one. Spirochaetes grow poorly on culture and the frequency of isolation from infected patients is low. Serological techniques include Western blotting and ELISA. 50% of early stage and 80% of late stage patients are seropositive.

Treatment is with antibiotics. Antibiotics used include penicillin, amoxil, erythromycin and ceftriaxone. The response to antibiotic therapy is generally good. Prognosis is excellent. 3–4% of children develop a chronic arthritis and a very small number have chronic neurological or cardiac sequelae.

163. PARVOVIRUS B19 INFECTION   Answer: ABCE

Parvovirus B19 is a DNA virus. Humans are the only host. Spread is by droplet. Infectivity is high (particularly before the rash appears). Infection is commonest in school age children but can occur at any age.

Infection with parvovirus B19 can be asymptomatic. More commonly it presents as erythema infectiosum, initially with mild fever and upper respiratory tract symptoms with the later appearance of a facial rash (slapped cheek syndrome). The rash usually spreads to the trunk and can persist for several days. Other manifestations of parvovirus B19 infection include purpura, lymphadenopathy and aplastic anaemia. The aplastic anaemia is usually temporary and is more common in children with either sickle cell disease or hereditary spherocytosis. Arthralgia/arthropathy is common in older patients, especially females.

In-utero infection is associated with spontaneous abortion, hydrops fetalis and neonatal thrombocytopenia.

The diagnosis of parvovirus infection is essentially a clinical one. The patient may be anaemic with a low reticulocyte count. The platelet count and white cell count may also be reduced. Anti-parvovirus IgM is the best marker of acute infection and is usually positive within 2 weeks of the onset of infection.

Treatment is essentially symptomatic. Intravenous immunoglobulin has been used in children with immunodeficiency and those with aplastic anaemia.

Differential diagnosis of parvovirus B19 infection
Rubella
Measles
Enterovirus infection
Drugs
Rash and arthropathy
    Juvenile chronic arthritis
    Systemic lupus erythematosus
    Other connective tissue disease

164. VERTICAL TRANSMISSION OF HEPATITIS B   Answer: ABDE

Vertical transmission is thought to account for 40% of hepatitis B world-wide. The hallmark of ongoing infection is the presence of HBsAg. The presence of antibody to HBsAg alone suggests successful immunisation; its presence along with anti-HBcAg suggests resolved infection.

Vertical transmission
This is mainly thought to occur around the time of birth. The risk of transmission is increased to >90% if the mother is hepatitis B 'e' antigen positive. Hepatitis B immunoglobulin given at birth alone reduces the risk of vertical transmission. The effect of giving active immunisation (hepatitis B vaccine at birth, 1 and 6 months) and passive immunisation with hepatitis B immunoglobulin is additive. Protection is achieved in 93% of neonates. Active immunisation does not seem to be affected by transmitted maternal IgG.

165. IRRITABLE HIP   Answer B

Transient synovitis of the hip
This occurs most commonly between the ages of 2 and 10 years. It affects boys more frequently than girls. The cause is uncertain; active or recent viral infection (70%), trauma and allergic hypersensitivity may play a role.

Investigations should include a full blood count, ESR and X-ray of the hip joint. The ultrasound may demonstrate a small effusion.

Transient synovitis of the hip resolves with bedrest, with or without traction within 7–10 days.

Septic arthritis
This can occur at any age, but it is commoner below 10 years. Children are usually pyrexial, toxic and unwell with a neutrophilia and raised ESR. X-rays can be normal initially. Aspiration of the joint is almost always necessary. Organisms include *Staphylococcus aureus, Haemophilus influenzae, E. Coli, Streptococcus, Salmonella* and *Meningococcus*. Blood cultures are positive in 50–70%. Management is with antibiotics for at least 3 weeks, pain relief and rehabilitative physiotherapy. Surgical drainage is often required.

166. VERTICAL TRANSMISSION OF HIV   Answer: ACE

Risk factors
Advanced clinical disease in the mother
Low CD4 count
Presence of other sexually transmitted diseases
Amnionitis
Prolonged rupture of membranes
Preterm delivery
Breast feeding

Caesarian section reduces the risk.

167. ERYTHEMA NODOSUM   Answer: ABCDE

Causes
Idiopathic
Streptococcal infection
Tuberculosis
Leptospirosis
Histoplasmosis
Epstein-Barr virus infection
Herpes simplex virus
Yersinia
Sulphonamides
Oral contraceptive pill
Systemic lupus erythematosus
Crohn's disease
Ulcerative colitis
Behçet's syndrome
Sarcoidosis
Hodgkin's disease

168. SYSTEMIC LUPUS ERYTHEMATOSUS (SLE)   **Answer: ACDE**

20% of SLE begins in childhood. There is a higher incidence in dark skinned racial groups. The female to male ratio is 8:1. HLA associations B8, DW2/DR3 and DW2/DR2. The onset can be insidious or acute. Early features usually include fever, malaise, arthralgia and a rash. There are many other manifestations and many organ systems can be involved. Treatment is with immunosuppression and anti-inflammatory agents.

Clinical features
Butterfly rash
Discoid rash
Erythematous macules
Nail changes
Erythema nodosum
Erythema multiforme
Arthritis and arthralgia
Polyserositis (pleuritis, pericarditis, peritonitis)
Cardiac including thrombosis and myocardial infarction
Pulmonary fibrosis
Renal (nephrotic syndrome, nephritis, chronic renal failure)
Gastrointestinal
Seizures
Psychosis

Laboratory features
Anaemia of chronic disease
Leucopenia
Thrombocytopenia
Coomb's positive haemolytic anaemia

Serology
Anti-nuclear antibody (ANA) should be present in all cases of active SLE, although there are other causes of ANA positivity (see later). There are different types of anti-nuclear antibody which are more specific.
- Ro/SSA and Lo/SSB present in neonatal lupus.
- Anti-DNA antibody which is specific for SLE and associated with renal involvement.
- Anti-Sm (soluble nuclear protein) antigen.

C3 is low in severe lupus and is a marker of disease activity. Anti-cardiolipin antibody is often present and reflects a thrombotic tendency.

Drug induced SLE
Certain drugs can induce SLE and ANA positivity and these include anticonvulsants, hydralazine, sulphonamides and procainamide. The disease tends to run a milder course. CNS and renal involvement are unusual.

Causes of ANA positivity in children
Juvenile chronic arthritis (particularly the pauciarticular type, ANA positivity associated with eye disease)
Chronic active hepatitis
Scleroderma
Mixed connective tissue disease
Drugs
Epstein-Barr virus infection

Causes of anti neutrophil cytoplasmic antibodies (ANCA)
Ulcerative colitis
Crescentic glomerulonephritis
Cholangitis
Chronic active hepatitis

169. PERTHES' DISEASE   Answer: AD

The pathology is of ischaemic necrosis of the femoral head involving the epiphysis and adjacent metaphysis. The process is initially a destructive one followed by regeneration.

The incidence is 1 in 2000. Age at presentation is between 2 and 10 years. The male to female ratio is 4:1. It usually occurs in isolation but can occur in association with congenital dislocation of the hip, mucopolysaccharidosis, achondroplasia and rickets. 10% of cases are bilateral. Diagnosis is by lateral X-ray of the appropriate hip joint.

Slipped upper femoral epiphysis
This is associated with obesity and microgenitalia. 20% are bilateral. It usually presents with knee and hip pain. Lateral X-ray of the hip is diagnostic. Complications include premature epiphyseal fusion and avascular necrosis.

170. IMMUNISATIONS	Answer: BD
171. IMMUNISATIONS	Answer: ABCE
172. IMMUNISATIONS	Answer: A

A thorough knowledge of immunisation is required and the reader is referred to the 1996 Handbook of Immunisation. Contraindications and indications to vaccination depend on the vaccine used and the medical condition of the child.

Immunocompromised individuals (e.g. congenital immune disorders, children on high dose corticosteroids or immunosuppressive therapy and children with malignancy or other tumours of the reticuloendothelial system) should not receive live vaccines. Live polio vaccine should not be given to siblings of immunocompromised individuals due to the risk of viral transmission, instead killed (Salk) poliovirus vaccine should be given.

HIV positive individuals with or without symptoms can receive MMR and polio live vaccines. They should not receive BCG, yellow fever or oral typhoid vaccines.

DTP vaccination is contraindicated if on previous exposure there has been seizures within 3 days of vaccine, encephalitis or collapse and shock (all associated with pertussis component). Reactions to pertussis vaccination are reduced in studies using the acellular pertussis vaccines rather than cellular pertussis vaccines.

MMR, influenza and yellow fever vaccines produced in chick embryos are contraindicated in children with a history of having had an anaphylactic reaction to egg. The most recent Handbook of Immunisation suggests that the MMR is probably safe even if the child has had an anaphylactic reaction to egg. Cases in which there is any concern should be immunised in hospital.

The most common side effects after MMR vaccination are fever and rash a week after vaccination. Parotid swelling occasionally occurs in the third week. The incidence of meningoencephalitis (rare, with complete recovery) has fallen since the change in the mumps vaccine component of MMR.

Live vaccines are ineffective up to 3–12 months after immunoglobulin infusions, they are also less effective if given within 3 weeks of a previous live vaccine.

Common side effects of BCG vaccination include localised skin ulceration, sterile abscess at injection site and regional adenitis. BCG vaccine should only be given after testing for hypersensitivity to tuberculoprotein, except in newborn infants where testing is not necessary before vaccine is given.

Influenza vaccines are recommended only for children at high risk e.g. chronic respiratory disease (including asthma, bronchopulmonary dysplasia and cystic fibrosis), chronic heart disease, chronic renal disease, diabetes mellitus and other endocrine disorders.

Pneumococcal vaccine is indicated in those at increased risk of pneumococcal infection e.g. sickle cell disease, asplenic patients, immunocompromised children (including HIV). It has minimal effect if given before the age of 2 years.

173. HLA B27 POSITIVITY   Answer: AC

Conditions associated with HLA B27 positivity
Ankylosing spondylitis
Reiter's syndrome
Arthritis of inflammatory bowel disease and psoriasis
Acute iridocyclitis
Pauciarticular arthritis of older children
Reactive arthritis following infection with *Salmonella, Shigella, Yersinia Enterocolitica, Campylobacter.*

Ankylosing spondylitis
95% of cases of ankylosing spondylitis are associated with HLA B27 positivity. Ankylosing spondylitis occurs predominantly in adolescence with an onset usually over the age of 8 years. The classical arthritis is of the sacroiliac joint and lower lumbar spine although other joints are involved, particularly in the early stages. 25% develop an acute iridocyclitis.

Reiter's syndrome
Reiter's syndrome classically comprises the triad of sterile urethritis, arthritis and ocular inflammation. Gastrointestinal symptoms and skin rashes also occur. Reiter's syndrome is commoner in males than in females. The arthritis is usually pauciarticular. It can occur following infection with *Shigella, Yersinia, Campylobacter* and *Chlamydia.*

Inflammatory bowel disease
10% of children with inflammatory bowel disease develop an arthritis. A number develop ankylosing spondylitis and this is associated with HLA B27 positivity.

Reactive arthritis
Reactive arthritis can occur following infection with *Salmonella*, *Shigella*, *Yersinia enterocolitica* and *Campylobacter pylori*. There is an HLA B27 association. The relationship between Reiter's syndrome and reactive arthritis is unclear.

Psoriatic arthritis
Psoriatic arthritis has a weak HLA B27 association. The arthritis itself is commoner in girls. It is asymmetrical. Nail pitting and distal interphalangeal joint involvement is common.

Neither Marfan's syndrome nor diabetes mellitus have an association with HLA B27 positivity. Dermatomyositosis is associated with HLA B8/DR3.

174. KAWASAKI'S DISEASE   Answer: CD

Kawasaki's disease is an acute, self limiting, systemic vasculitis of unknown aetiology that affects infants and young children. The vasculitis involves medium and small vessels.

Clinical and epidemiological characteristics suggest toxin-induced superantigen stimulation. Person-to-person transmission has not been documented.

Diagnostic criteria for Kawasaki's disease
Fever persisting for 5 days or more
Four of the following:
    Bilateral non-suppurative conjunctivitis
    Polymorphous exanthema
    Cervical lymphadenopathy
    Inflammation of the tongue, lips and oral mucosa
    Oedema and erythema of the hands and feet
Illness not explained by a known disease process

Atypical Kawasaki's disease implies that not all the diagnostic criteria are met but clinically the child is felt to have Kawasaki's disease and later coronary artery dilatation or other pathognomonic criteria develop. Atypical Kawasaki's disease is commoner in infants than in older children. Infants have a higher incidence of coronary artery aneurysms.

There are three stages of the disease, acute, subacute and convalescent. The acute stage lasts 0–2 weeks and comprises fever, conjunctivitis, oral changes, irritability, rash and lymphadenopathy. The subacute stage lasts for 21 days and is when skin peeling, thrombocytosis and coronary artery aneurysms occur. Symptoms resolve during the convalescent phase. There is usually a leucocytosis, raised CRP, raised ESR and a transient disturbance of liver function in the acute stage. Thrombocytosis occurs later. These abnormalities resolve during the convalescent phase.

The major complications are cardiac with the development of coronary artery aneurysms which occur in 10–40% of untreated patients. The majority of patients do well, however 1–2% die of cardiac complications e.g. myocardial ischaemia.

Treatment is with intravenous immunoglobulin administered within the first 10 days of the illness at a dose of 2 g/kg. This is associated with a reduction in symptoms and the incidence of coronary artery aneurysms. Aspirin is also used for its anti-inflammatory and anti-platelet effects. A high dose of 100 mg/kg is used in the acute phase with a maintenance dose of 5 mg/kg/day in the convalescent phase. All children in whom the diagnosis of Kawasaki's disease is suspected should be referred for an echocardiogram.

175. RUBELLA
Answer: BCDE

Transmission of rubella is by droplet spread. The incubation period is 14–21 days. Infection can be asymptomatic. Infection is now rare as a consequence of the immunisation programme.

Prodromal symptoms may or may not be present and precede the rash by 1–5 days. These include fever, coryza, conjunctivitis and lymphadenopathy (sub-occipital, post auricular and cervical). The rash is macular and lasts for 3–5 days.

Complications include persistent lymphadenopathy, arthritis, neuritis, thrombocytopenic purpura and encephalitis (associated with a CSF lymphocytosis).

Differential diagnosis of rubella
Infectious mononucleosis
Toxoplasmosis
Enteroviral infection
Roseola, scarlet fever
Mycoplasma
Parvovirus infection

Viral isolation is difficult and diagnosis is by serology. Treatment is supportive. Prevention is by immunisation with the MMR vaccine.

Congenital rubella occurs secondary to maternal infection in the first trimester. Clinical manifestations are variable and include:
• Jaundice
• Thrombocytopenia
• Growth retardation
• Cardiac abnormalities
• Eye problems (cataracts, blindness, microphthalmia)
• Deafness
• Microcephaly
• Fetal death
• Stillbirth

176. ASSESSMENT OF GESTATIONAL AGE   Answer: BDE

Gestational age assessment is usually done by calculation from the first day of the mother's last menstrual period or an early ultrasound. Gestational age can be estimated after birth by careful physical and neurological examination. This needs to be done on the first day as some signs change rapidly after birth.

Physical signs used include:
- skin colour, texture and opacity
- lanugo hair
- plantar creases
- oedema of the feet and hands
- ear form and firmness
- breast size
- nipple formation
- genital appearance

Neurological criteria depend on muscle tone (decreased in preterms) and joint mobility (increases with gestational age).

The scarf sign refers to when the arm is pulled across the supine infant to wrap it around the opposite shoulder. The elbow reaches the opposite axilla in very preterm infants but does not reach the midline in term infants.

177. PERSISTENT FETAL CIRCULATION   Answer: ABE

Persistent fetal circulation (persistent pulmonary hypertension of the newborn) is characterised by hypoxia which is out of proportion to the severity of lung disease, a structurally normal heart and evidence of right to left shunting either at the ductus or through the foramen ovale. Echocardiography is the investigation of choice to confirm the diagnosis.

Risk factors include birth asphyxia, group B streptococcal sepsis, pulmonary hypoplasia (diaphragmatic hernia, oligohydramnios, pleural effusion), meconium aspiration syndrome, hyaline membrane disease, maternal indomethacin and high pressure ventilation.

Management includes minimal handling, maintenance of a normal arterial blood pressure, normalisation of acid base status and broad spectrum antibiotics. Hyperventilation, by driving down the $PaCO_2$ causes vasodilation and a rise in PaO_2.

Tolazoline dilates both the pulmonary and systemic circulation. It is best infused through a central line direct into the right atrium. The systemic vasodilation means that colloid support often needs to be given concurrently. Other pulmonary vasodilators include magnesium sulphate, prostacyclin and nitric oxide. Other therapeutic approaches include high frequency oscillatory ventilation and extracorporeal membrane oxygenation (ECMO).

Extracorporeal membrane oxygenation (ECMO)
Extracorporeal membrane oxygenation (ECMO) is a form of cardiopulmonary bypass that allows gas exchange outside the body and increases systemic perfusion. It is commonly performed as veno-arterial ECMO (right internal jugular to carotid). Blood pumped into the circuit is oxygenated by a membrane oxygenator and returned. Veno-venous ECMO allows gas exchange but does not support the cardiac output.

178. AIR LEAK SYNDROME IN THE NEWBORN   Answer: E

A pneumothorax is present in approximately 1% of newborns (the quoted figure is very variable) and is usually asymptomatic.

Risk factors for pneumothorax
Respiratory distress syndrome
Active resuscitation
Meconium aspiration
Pulmonary hypoplasia

Risk factors in ventilated babies
High peak pressure and mean airway pressure
High positive end expiratory pressure
Prolonged inspiratory time
Increased I:E ratios
Inadequate sedation (controversial)

Asymptomatic pneumothoraces or pneumothoraces causing only minor symptoms in term babies can be treated with 100% oxygen to hasten absorption by decreasing the partial pressure of nitrogen in the blood which increases the absorption of nitrogen from the pneumothorax.

Insertion of an underwater seal drain is indicated in all infants with moderate or severe symptoms and in virtually all ventilated babies with a pneumothorax regardless of whether or not the pneumothorax is under tension.

Pneumomediastinum, pneumopericardium and pneumoperitoneum can all be asymptomatic. However all can be responsible for an acute deterioration in the clinical state of a ventilated baby. A pneumopericardium can cause acute cardiac tamponade.

179. SMALL FOR GESTATIONAL AGE INFANTS   Answer: ABCD

An infant is considered small for dates or small for gestational age if its birth weight is less than 2 standard deviations below the mean for its gestational age. There are many causes of this. These can be maternal, fetal and placental. Small for gestational age infants can be symmetrically or asymmetrically growth retarded. Asymmetric growth retardation (head growth spared) is most common. Symmetrical growth retardation occurs secondary to an insult early in pregnancy such as an intrauterine infection in the first trimester.

Causes of infants being born small for gestational age
Maternal   physiological – maternal height, age <20 or >35, multiparity
            pathological – toxaemia, hypertension, smoking,
            alcoholism, malnutrition, chronic disease
Fetal   physiological – genetic potential, multiple pregnancy,
            female sex
            pathological – chromosomal, infection, syndromal
            Placental infarction, tumour, feto-fetal transfusion, placental
            abruption

Problems of small for gestational age infants
Perinatal asphyxia
Meconium aspiration syndrome
Hypothermia
Hypoglycaemia
Polycythaemia
Heart failure
Persistent fetal circulation
Pulmonary haemorrhage
Increased risk of infection
Necrotising enterocolitis
Dysmorphology

Retrolental fibroplasia is a sequelae of retinopathy of prematurity which occurs in preterm infants, usually only those born below 32 weeks' gestation.

180. STEROID THERAPY IN THE NEWBORN   Answer: CDE

Steroids are indicated in ventilator-dependent preterm babies. They are initiated in order to reduce ventilator requirements and so reduce barotrauma from ventilation. They are usually started if a baby remains ventilator-dependent at 28 days although many units start treatment much earlier.

Proposed mechanisms of action
Stabilisation of membranes
Reduction in pulmonary oedema
Increased surfactant synthesis
Reduction of airway inflammation
Relief of bronchospasm

Side effects
Hypertension
Gastrointestinal bleeding
Gastric perforation
Hyperglycaemia
Sepsis
Cataracts
Cardiomyopathy
Leucocytosis

181. NECROTISING ENTEROCOLITIS   Answer: ACE

Necrotising enterocolitis is a condition of unknown aetiology most common in infants below 1500 g and characterised by transmural intestinal necrosis.

Predisposing factors
Hypoxia
Hypotension
Prematurity
Small for dates
Birth asphyxia
Hypothermia

Exchange transfusion/umbilical catheterisation
Polycythaemia
Formula feeding/rapidly increasing enteral feeding in preterms
Hypertonic feeds

Necrotising enterocolitis can occur in outbreaks. In less than 50% is an organism isolated. Organisms isolated include *E. Coli*, *Staphylococcus epidermidis*, rotavirus and *Clostridium perfingens*. *Clostridium welchii* causes gas gangrene.

Medical treatment consists of nil by mouth with nasogastric decompression, total parenteral nutrition and intravenous antibiotics. Ventilatory support is often required. Patients require regular monitoring (clinical, haematological, biochemical and radiological). Infants with Necrotising enterocolitis that fail to respond to medical therapy need to be assessed by a paediatric surgeon. The indications for surgery include perforation of the bowel, persistent bowel obstruction, presence of a fixed mass and continued deterioration despite medical therapy.

Late complications of necrotising enterocolitis include
• stricture formation
• short bowel syndrome
• blind loop syndrome
• cholestasis
• fistula
• cyst formation
• polyposis.

182. BIRTH INJURIES   Answer: ACE

Fractures are said to occur in up to 1% of infants at the time of their birth with clavicular fractures being the most common. Risk factors include shoulder dystocia and breech delivery.

Injury to the cervical spine is rare but can occur (with or without X-ray changes). Excessive rotation during cephalic deliveries results in injury at C1-2 level and breech deliveries with excessive traction result in damage at C6-T1. Hypotonia, hyporeflexia and hypoventilation ensue. MRI is useful for diagnosis.

Brachial plexus injuries usually result from traction injury during the delivery of infants with shoulder dystocia.

- Upper brachial plexus, Erb-Duchenne paralysis (C5-6). Affected arm is held in the waiter's tip position. Biceps and supinator reflexes are absent. Hand grasp is preserved. Diaphragmatic involvement can cause paradoxical movement of the chest wall on the affected side.
- Lower brachial plexus injury, Klumpke's paralysis (C8-T1), claw hand deformity, absent triceps jerk and palmar grasp with sometimes an ipsilateral Horner's syndrome.
- Total brachial plexus injury, Erb-Duchenne-Klumpke, combines features of both.

There are important differences between caput succedaneum (oedema over the presenting part of the scalp) and cephalohaematoma (haematoma between the skull and periosteum).

Caput succedaneum	Cephalohaematoma
Diffuse, ecchymotic, oedematous overlying skin	Normal overlying skin
Present at birth	Not present until a few hours after birth
Disappears over a few days	Reabsorbed over 2 weeks to 3 months Can calcify
May extend over suture lines	Limited by suture lines
No treatment needed	May require phototherapy for jaundice

183. RECURRENT APNOEA IN PRETERMS   Answer: ABCDE

Apnoea is a common symptom is preterm babies. Apnoea can be primary (recurrent apnoea of prematurity) or secondary to other phenomena.

Causes of secondary apnoea
Infection
Gastrointestinal tract – overfeeding, passage of stool, gastro-oesophageal reflux
Metabolic – hypoglycaemia, hypernatraemia, hyponatraemia
Cardiovascular – hypotension, fluid overload, heart failure
Respiratory – hypoxia, pneumonia, respiratory distress syndrome
Nervous system – haemorrhage, birth asphyxia, drugs

Apnoea with no underlying cause is apneoa of prematurity. This usually presents in preterms within a few days of birth and disappears by about 34 weeks' gestation. Many factors are thought to have a role in the pathogenesis including immaturity of the respiratory centre, upper airway collapse, environmental temperature and sleep state. Apnoea of prematurity is usually treated with a respiratory stimulant such as caffeine or theophylline.

184. RESPIRATORY DISTRESS SYNDROME   Answer: ABC

Respiratory distress syndrome (hyaline membrane disease) accounts for 30% of all neonatal deaths. The incidence is directly proportional to gestation. It is due to immaturity of the enzyme systems required to synthesise surfactant in the type 2 alveolar cells. Deficient surfactant on the alveolar surface results in high surface tension and atelectasis. This results in decreased lung compliance and a failure to establish a functional residual capacity. The major components of surfactant are dipalmitoyl phosphatidyl choline (lecithin), phosphatidyl glycerol, apolipoproteins (surfactant proteins SP-A, B,C,D) and cholesterol.

Factors that increase the risk of respiratory distress syndrome
Prematurity
Male sex
Twin pregnancy
Caesarian section
Hypothermia
Hypoglycaemia
Birth asphyxia
Maternal diabetes

Antenatal steroids administered to the mother 48–72 hours before delivery will reduce the incidence of respiratory distress syndrome.

Surfactant, which can be natural (survanta, curosurf) or synthetic (exosurf, ALEC) is administered to ventilated preterm infants either prophylactically (soon after birth) or as rescue when symptoms develop. Surfactant reduces the severity and the mortality from respiratory distress syndrome but not the incidence of bronchopulmonary dysplasia.

Other causes of respiratory distress in preterms
Transient tachypnoea of the newborn
Meconium aspiration syndrome
Birth asphyxia
Pulmonary haemorrhage
Sepsis including congenital pneumonia
Pneumothorax

Congenital abnormality – diaphragmatic hernia, tracheo-oesophageal fistula
Persistent fetal circulation
Congenital heart disease
Congenital lung cyst / congenital lobar emphysema
Pulmonary hypoplasia

185. PHOTOTHERAPY   Answer: ADE

Phototherapy reduces serum unconjugated bilirubin levels. It uses light at a wavelength of 420–550 nm in the blue green spectrum and causes bilirubin to become water soluble which allows excretion without conjugation.

It is indicated for the treatment of infants with pathological unconjugated hyperbilirubinaemia and is sometimes used prophylactically in very low birth weight babies. It reduces the need for exchange transfusion in infants with hyperbilirubinaemia, but when the indications for exchange exist it is not a substitute.

There is no absolute consensus as to the level at which phototherapy should be started although there are a number of charts which are widely used. Phototherapy is continued until the unconjugated bilirubin drops to safe levels. Colour of the skin does not alter its efficacy.

Rebound hyperbilirubinaemia usually occurs after stopping photo-therapy. Skin colour is inaccurate as a method of assessment of the bilirubin level of infants who are under phototherapy.

Infants' eyes should be covered while they are under phototherapy. Complications of phototherapy include loose stools, rash, dehydration, hypothermia, reduced mother–infant bonding.

186. INFANTS OF DIABETIC MOTHERS   Answer: CDE

Clinical features
General
    Macrosomia
    Normal head size
    Increased subcutaneous fat
    Birth trauma
CNS
    Jitteriness

Hyperexcitability
Hypotonia
Lethargy
Convulsions
Respiratory distress syndrome
Cardiovascular
Cardiomegaly (30%)
Transient hypertrophic cardiomyopathy
Persistent fetal circulation
Renal vein thrombosis
Metabolic
Hypoglycaemia (usually within the first few hours)
Hypocalcaemia
Hypomagnesaemia
Hyperbilirubinaemia
Haemotological
Polycythaemia
Congenital malformations – (3 fold increase)
Cardiac (ventricular septal defect, atrio ventricular septal defect, transposition of the great arteries, coarctation of the aorta)
Neural tube defects
Holoprosencephaly
Sacral agenesis
Hydronephrosis
Renal agenesis
Duodenal atresia
Anorectal malformations
Microcolon
Increased risk of diabetes mellitus

187. NEONATAL POLYCYTHAEMIA   Answer: BC

Polycythaemia refers to a raised haematocrit (packed cell volume). Neonatal polycythaemia is usually said to be present if the venous packed cell volume is greater than 65%.

Predisposing factors
Post maturity
Small for gestational age
Delayed cord clamping
Feto-fetal transfusion
Beckwith-Wiedemann syndrome

Infant of a diabetic mother
13/18/21 trisomy
Adrenogenital syndrome
Hypothyroidism
High altitude

Clinical features/complications
Respiratory – tachypnoea, respiratory distress, persistent fetal circulation
Cardiovascular system – heart failure
Gastrointestinal – feeding problems, vomiting, necrotising enterocolitis
Renal – renal vein thrombosis
Nervous system – lethargy, hypotonia, seizures, irritability
Skin – plethora
Haematological – thrombocytopenia
Biochemical – hypoglycaemia, hypocalcaemia, hyperbilirubinaemia

Treatment of polycythaemia includes ensuring an adequate fluid intake and attention to predisposing factors. Symptomatic infants may require a partial exchange transfusion of blood for either fresh frozen plasma or human albumin. The indications for this are controversial. Consideration of exchange should be in those infants who are symptomatic with a packed cell volume greater than 65% or those who have a packed cell volume greater than 70%. Late neurological sequelae are seen in some infants with symptomatic polycythaemia.

188. PERINATAL ASPHYXIA   Answer: ACE

Risk factors for perinatal asphyxia can be maternal, fetal or placental. Examples include
• Maternal – amnionitis, toxaemia, diabetes, smoking
• Placental – insufficiency, abruption
• Fetal – multiple gestation, small for dates, preterm gestation, congenital abnormalities

Effects of asphyxia
Respiratory – persistent fetal circulation, pulmonary haemorrhage, surfactant deficiency
Cardiovascular – myocardial ischaemia and heart failure, hypotension
CNS – hypoxic ischaemic encephalopathy, intracranial haemorrhage, cerebral oedema, cerebral infarction (periventricular leucomalacia)
Renal – acute tubular necrosis, adrenal haemorrhage
Gastrointestinal – perforation, ulceration, necrotising enterocolitis

Metabolic – hyponatraemia (inappropriate antidiuretic hormone secretion), hypoglycaemia, hypocalcaemia
Haematological – disseminated intravascular coagulation, haemorrhage

Hypoxic ischaemic encephalopathy is graded as follows:
- Grade I – irritability, hypotonia, poor suck, no seizures
- Grade II – lethargy, abnormal tone, requirement for tube feeds, seizures
- Grade III – comatose, severe hypotonia, failure to maintain respiration without respiratory support, prolonged seizures

Less than 10% of cerebral palsy is as a consequence of perinatal asphyxia.

189. BILE STAINED VOMITING   Answer: E

Duodenal atresia
This accounts for 25–40% of all intestinal atresias. Half are preterm and 20–30% have Down's syndrome. Malrotation, oesophageal atresia, anorectal malformations and congenital heart disease are associated abnormalities. Bilious vomiting with abdominal distension on day one is common. Visible gastric peristalsis can occur.

Pyloric stenosis
Multifactorial inheritance. Projectile non-bilious vomiting, onset between 3 weeks and 5 months. Infant presents hungry and with weight loss. First born males are more commonly affected. Palpable pyloric tumour and visible gastric peristalsis present. Mild unconjugated hyperbilirubin-aemia and hypochloraemic, hypokalaemic metabolic alkalosis occur. Ultrasound confirms the diagnosis.
Treatment is by pyloromyotomy (Ramstedt's procedure) after correction of the electrolyte and acid base disturbance.

Malrotation
This refers to incomplete rotation of the mid gut during fetal development. This results in the small bowel occupying the right side of the abdomen and the large bowel the left. The caecum is often sub-hepatic. The mesentery along with the superior mesenteric artery is attached by a narrow stalk which can twist around itself producing a mid gut volvulus. Infants can present with bile stained vomiting and abdominal distension in the first few weeks or later with episodes of abdominal colic and vomiting. Diagnosis is by barium meal and follow

through. Barium enema may show a malpositioned caecum but is not the investigation of choice.

Meconium can still be passed with obstruction of the upper small bowel. Meconium ileus occurs in cystic fibrosis and is the presenting feature in 10%. Presentation is in the neonatal period with failure to pass meconium and abdominal distension. Treatment is with gastrograffin enemas. Up to 50% require surgery.

190. NEONATAL HAEMATOLOGY   Answer: CE

Cord haemoglobin levels in term infants range from 14–20 g/dl. The levels in preterms are lower. Over the first few months a physiological anaemia occurs. This is due to reduced red cell survival, relative hyperoxia and increasing blood volume due to increasing weight.

Anaemia at birth is most commonly due to immune haemolysis. The other main cause is acute blood loss. Anaemia due to reduced red cell production is not usually noticed till 3–4 weeks of age.

Fetal haemoglobin constitutes 70% of the haemoglobin at birth. It contains two alpha and two gamma chains.

Alpha thalassaemia may present in the neonatal period. Beta thalassaemia does not.

Fetal haemoglobin is resistant to alkaline denaturation unlike adult haemoglobin; this is the basis of the Apt test used to differentiate fetal blood from swallowed maternal blood in the gut (for example on a gastric aspirate).

Causes of anaemia in the neonate
Blood loss
    Placental abruption
    Feto-fetal haemorrhage
    Feto-maternal bleed
    Cephalhaematoma
    Intraventricular haemorrhage
    Iatrogenic – surgical, frequent sampling, snapped cord at delivery
Haemolysis
    ABO incompatibility
    Rhesus disease

Hereditary spherocytosis
G6PD deficiency
Impaired production
    Pure red cell aplasia – Diamond-Blackfan syndrome

191. PROBLEMS ASSOCIATED WITH PRETERM GESTATION

Answer: ABCDE

There are many problems associated with preterm gestation. A number are listed below. Details of these problems should be learnt and can be found in any of the pocket books of neonatal intensive care (see bibliography).

Respiratory distress syndrome
Pneumothorax
Chronic lung disease
Hypotension
Patent ductus arteriosus
Hyponatraemia
Hypernatraemia
Glycosuria
Hypoglycaemia
Hyperglycaemia
Hyperbilirubinaemia
Intraventricular haemorrhage
Periventricular leucomalacia
Retinopathy of prematurity
Anaemia
Infection
Necrotising enterocolitis
Apnoea of prematurity

192. NEONATAL FITS

Answer: BCE

Causes
Hypoxic ischaemic encephalopathy
Intraventricular haemorrhage
Meningitis
Hypoglycaemia
Hypocalcaemia
Hyponatraemia
Hypernatraemia

Inborn error of metabolism
Kernicterus
Fifth day fits
Drug withdrawal
Congenital malformation
Idiopathic

Both Wilson's disease and lead poisoning would present outside the neonatal period.

Di George's syndrome can present with hypocalcaemia. Other causes of hypocalcaemia in the neonatal period include maternal vitamin D deficiency, high phosphate milks, renal failure, primary hypoparathyroidism, maternal hyperparathyroidism and hypomagnesaemia.

193. CONGENITAL DISLOCATION OF THE HIP   Answer: ABDE

Risk factors for congenital dislocation of the hip
Family history (positive in 20%)
Female sex (female:male, 6:1)
Breech delivery (factor in 30%)
Spina bifida
Being first born
Oligohydramnios

The left hip is more likely to be dislocated than the right. Ultrasound is the best test for diagnosis. The clinical tests of hip instability are Ortolani's and Barlow's.

194. CAUSES OF CONJUGATED   Answer: CDE
HYPERBILIRUBINAEMIA IN THE NEONATAL PERIOD

Infectious – hepatitis A, B, C, cytomegalovirus, rubella, herpes simplex
Metabolic – cystic fibrosis, tyrosinaemia, galactosaemia, fructosaemia
Intrahepatic – Alagille's syndrome, congenital hepatic fibrosis
Extrahepatic – biliary atresia, choledochal cyst, inspissated bile
         syndrome
Toxic – total parenteral nutrition related, sepsis, urinary tract infection,
         drugs
Endocrine – hypopituitarism, hypothyroidism
Miscellaneous – intestinal obstruction

All infants with prolonged neonatal jaundice (greater than 2 weeks) need investigation.

Infants with a predominantly conjugated hyperbilirubinaemia require referral for investigation in a liver unit, particularly to exclude biliary atresia which has a much better outcome if surgery (Kasai procedure) is performed within the first 8 weeks.

195. CHICKENPOX   Answer: BC

Children born to mothers who develop chickenpox during the period 7 days before delivery and 7 days after should be given varicella zoster immunoglobulin (ZIG). Breast feeding should be encouraged and any baby who develops chickenpox lesions should be treated with i.v. aciclovir. Untreated the mortality is around 30%.

ZIG should probably be offered to infants exposed to chickenpox during the neonatal period (i.e. up to 4 weeks of age). This is not always possible as ZIG is in short supply – refer to Department of Health: Immunisation against Infectious Disease (1996).

If a mother develops chickenpox during the first trimester then the infant is at risk of developing congenital varicella syndrome, the risk being 1–2%. The congenital varicella syndrome includes limb hypoplasia, microcephaly, cataract, growth retardation, and skin scarring.

COMMUNITY PAEDIATRICS AND CHILD PSYCHIATRY ANSWERS

196. ANOREXIA NERVOSA

Answer: ABD

The characteristic features of anorexia nervosa are severe weight loss, excessive exercising, depression (in about 50%), self-induced vomiting and laxative abuse associated with a distorted self image and a morbid fear of being fat.

It is more common in pubertal girls, in whom amennorhoea is usually present, than in pre-pubertal girls. The incidence is higher in pupils of fee-paying schools and children of higher socio-economic status. It is also higher in certain populations such as ballet dancers and fashion students. Concordance is greater in monozygotic than dizygotic twins.

The prevalence of anorexia is 0.5–1.0%. 1 in 10 cases are boys. 50% make a complete recovery, 25% make a partial recovery with some residual minor eating problems and the other 25% persist with a chronic course of illness. Mortality is 5%.

Bulimia nervosa

Bulimia nervosa is characterised by binge eating followed by self-induced vomiting and laxative abuse. They are not usually underweight but share the same fear as sufferers of anorexia nervosa of becoming fat. Dental caries is common.

197. AUTISM

Answer: AE

Autism usually presents before 3 years of age and is characterised by speech delay, absence of pretend play, stereotyped repetitive behaviour, lack of social interest and poor social interactions with parents and other children. The disorder is a spectrum and often called autistic spectrum disorder.

The incidence is 2–13 per 10 000. Boys are more commonly affected than girls by 3:1. There is a genetic association with 3% of siblings being affected.

One in five cases are associated with a medical condition, fragile X syndrome and tuberous sclerosis being the commonest. Mental retardation is common, 70% have an IQ <70. The more severe the mental retardation the more likely the child will have epilepsy in adolescence (20–30%). There is no association with social class or poor parenting.

50% gain useful language by 5 years of age but there is odd use of language with delayed echolalia and stereotyped phraseology. Useful acquisition of language by the age of 5 years is a good prognostic indicator for function in adult life. Two-thirds of autistics grow up to be severely handicapped adults, unable to look after themselves.

Asperger's syndrome
This is probably part of the autistic spectrum but a milder form with relatively normal IQ and language development. The prevalence is around 10–25 per 10,000. It is commoner in boys. Recognised personality traits include abnormalities of gaze, poverty of expression and gesture, unusual and narrow focus of intellectual interests and a lack of feeling for others. Most people with Asperger's are also clumsy.

198. HYPERKINETIC DISORDER   Answer: BCDE

Hyperactivity in childhood is common but is considered a disorder when it interferes with social function, learning and development. It is characterised by inattention, overactivity and impulsiveness. It affects 1 in 200 children. It is commoner in boys than girls, ratio 3 to 1.

Inattention leads to brief interest in activities and problems with learning and development. Overactivity is the excess of movements with restlessness and fidgeting. Impulsiveness causes action without thinking, often acting dangerously leading to frequent accidents. Behavioural therapy can lead to improvement but it is intensive.

Drug therapy is with stimulant drugs such as dexamphetamine and methylphenidate. Their use is controversial. Side effects of drug therapy are common and include insomnia, suppression of appetite and depression. Rare side effects include psychosis, growth retardation, increased frequency of tics and worsening of epilepsy. Modification of diet has been reported to improve symptoms in a number of children.

Assessment of symptoms and effect of treatment can be aided by use of the Connor Teacher's Rating Scale questionnaire to assess activity and attention at school.

Hyperkinetic disorder is associated, in adolescence, with increased risk of school expulsion, conduct disorder and increased risk of multiple accidents.

Some causes of hyperactivity in children
Normal variant
Understimulation/boredom
Learning difficulties
Autism
Temporal lobe epilepsy
Drugs e.g. anti-epileptic medication

199. SCHOOL REFUSAL   Answer: ABCD

School refusal is due to an excessive degree of anxiety making it difficult for the child to attend school. It occurs in about 1–2% of children of school age. There is equal sex incidence. It is commonest at age 5–6 years and 11 years when a new school is started. Depression is present in about 50–70%. Physical symptoms are common.

The outcome is very good with a programme of psychotherapy and flooding therapy (taking the child to school, often under supervision of the therapist). Drug therapy is not indicated in most cases, but tricyclic antidepressants, e.g. imipramine, have been shown to be of use when there is co-existent depression.

Truancy is differentiated from school refusal as it is the wilful avoidance of school and not due to anxiety about school attendance.

200. SQUINT   Answer: ABC

Childhood squint (strabismus) is the misalignment of the eyes during visual fixation. It is common in childhood affecting 4% of children <6 years. If left untreated it can cause secondary visual loss (amblyopia) in the affected eye.
Squint is divided into two categories
• Non-paralytic squint: where there is no abnormality of the extraocular muscles or nerves supplying them.
• Paralytic squint: where there is a weakness of one or more of the extra-ocular muscles leading to squint. This is less common and when it presents a cause must be sought.

Diagnosis
Corneal light reflex test. The degree of squint can be assessed using prisms in front of the eye while doing the test (Krimsky method).
Cover testing.

Visual acuity testing: this is mandatory to assess vision in both eyes.
Eye movements

Treatment of non-paralytic squint
Correction of any refractive error.
Patching the normal eye allowing the development of vision in the affected eye.
Corrective surgery. This is largely cosmetic and involves strengthening or weakening the appropriate extra-ocular muscles to balance out the squint. Often a second operation is required to align the eyes fully.

201. DEAFNESS
Answer: ADE

Deafness is either conductive, sensorineural or mixed. There are many causes of deafness and these should be learned. A number of causes are listed below,

Congenital
Autosomal dominant 33%
Autosomal recessive 65%
X linked 2%

Syndromes
Alport's syndrome (with renal failure)
Treacher-Collins syndrome
Klippel-Feil anomalies of the spine
Down's syndrome
Waardenberg's syndrome
Jervill-Lange-Nielson syndrome associated with prolonged QT interval and sudden death.
Pendred syndrome

Acquired
Pre-natal
    Congenital infection – rubella, cytomegalovirus
    Drugs such as thalidomide
Perinatal
    It is common in pre-term infants with a prevalence in very low birth weight infants (<1500g) of 1%. Pre-term infants are particularly susceptible to hypoxia, hyperbilirubinaemia, intra-ventricular haemorrhage and the use of drugs such as gentamicin.

Older children
  Otitis media
  Glue ear
  Meningitis

Assessment of deafness

- Oto-acoustic emissions: these are emitted by normal ears in response to sound emitted by an aural probe. They are not emitted by ears with a hearing loss of >30 dB, and it is an all or nothing response. They have a 100% sensitivity and 80% specificity for sensorineural hearing loss.
- Brain stem evoked auditory responses: electrodes are placed over the skull and electrical activity is picked up in response to auditory stimulation. This is a useful test in babies under 6 months of age especially in those at high risk of deafness (jaundice, prematurity, low birth weight). The test is not affected by sedation.
- Distraction testing is used from 6 months to 1 year of age.
- Play audiometry can be used after 18 months to 2 years of age.
- Pure tone audiometry is used after 3.5 years of age as this is the age in which co-operation can be achieved.

Glue ear

This is the commonest form of deafness in children. Causes include acute otitis media, allergy and malformation of the eustachian tube (associated with cleft palate). These all lead to accumulation of fluid in the middle ear which may become infected. The fluid prevents equalisation of pressures between the middle ear and the atmosphere from occurring and damps the response of the ear drum to sound. A large proportion of cases resolve spontaneously or with a trial of decongestant therapy. If not, treatment is with grommet insertion. The main indications are speech delay and severe hearing loss.

202. MUNCHAUSEN'S BY PROXY   Answer: ABCDE

Munchausen's by proxy, or factitious disease in childhood, is a disorder which can end with disability or even death. It involves fabrication of the child's symptoms by the parent or care giver and simulation of physical signs. Clinical presentations include:
- Poisoning
- Drug ingestion or injection
- Causing apnoeas by suffocation
- Physical injuries

Often the parent has a background in health care, presents as a good parent, gets on well with medical staff and seems to be unconcerned about their child's symptoms. The parent may also interfere with ward investigations (blood in stool or urine samples, diluting urine, altering the temperature measurements).

The diagnosis is often difficult to make but clues include:
- A persistent or recurrent illness which cannot be explained
- Investigation results that do not correlate with the health of the child
- Symptoms which do not occur while the parent is away
- The parent may not leave the child's bedside in hospital, even for short periods of time
- Treatment is ineffective or poorly tolerated, even if appropriate for the suspected clinical problem
- Inconsistent medical history

Investigation depends on symptomatology. Samples should be collected by medical staff to prevent contamination. Covert video surveillance has been used successfully in a number of cases of apnoea caused by parental suffocation.

Treatment involves protecting the child and siblings from potential harm. Involvement of social services at an early stage is essential.

203. INDICATIONS FOR REFERRAL TO A CHILD PSYCHIATRIST   Answer: ACE

- Emotional or behavioural problems unresponsive to first-line counselling
- Deliberate drug overdose or attempted suicide
- Difficult child protection cases
- Difficult diagnostic problems where there is no obvious organic cause.

Included in behavioural problems are those which are common in childhood
- Separation anxiety
- Soiling
- Persistent grief reactions
- Grief reactions causing severe disruption to the child or family environment.

A persistent grief reaction is one which has persisted beyond the normal age range. A general rule of thumb is that it is persistent if it lasts longer in months than the child's age in years.

Prevalence of psychiatric disorders in childhood
The prevalence of psychiatric disorder in childhood depends on the age range, the population studied and the diagnostic criteria used, however:
- Prevalence is higher in urban than rural areas.
- Conduct and hyperactivity disorders are commoner in boys at all ages.
- Emotional disorders show an equal sex distribution in 4–11 year olds, but are 3 times commoner in girls between the ages of 12–16 years.

Risk factors and associations of psychiatric disorder
Child
>   Severe learning disability, up to 40%
>   Low self-esteem and academic failure
>   Physical illness: strong association with epilepsy and slight increase in most other illnesses
>   Specific developmental delay, for example speech delay
>   Bullying and peer group pressure
>   Abuse

Family
>   Family breakdown (up to 80% incidence in children 1 year after divorce)
>   Maternal ill health
>   Paternal criminality, alcoholism
>   Abuse
>   Poverty
>   Death and loss, including loss of friendships
>   Inconsistent discipline
>   Family history of psychiatric disorder

204. CHILDHOOD DEPRESSION   Answer: BD

Major depressive illness in children is uncommon (2 per 1000), but many children have depressive symptoms and the incidence of both increase during adolescence. Depression can be primary (isolated depression) or secondary (secondary to other psychiatric disorder or physical disease).
- Primary depression is often associated with a family history of depression.
- Pre-pubertal boys are twice as likely to have depression as pre-pubertal girls. This sex incidence is reversed after puberty.

- Suicidal behaviour (parasuicide) is common in children who suffer from depression.
- Successful suicide in childhood is extremely rare.

Symptoms characteristically include depressed mood and tearfulness, lethargy and loss of interest in usual activities, feelings of guilt and self-blame, diminished appetite and poor weight gain (but appetite can be increased), impaired sleep (but can be increased), social withdrawal, outbursts of aggression and delusional symptoms in the form of auditory hallucinations accusing the child of worthlessness.

205. SUDDEN INFANT DEATH SYNDROME (SIDS)   Answer: AD

Sudden infant death is the unexpected and unexplained death of an infant (on post-mortem findings and on examination of the scene of death). The peak incidence is between 2–4 months of age with 95% of deaths occurring before 6 months of age. The incidence has been declining since 1989 when there were 1337 deaths, to 442 deaths in 1993. The incidence started declining before the government Back to Sleep campaign in 1991 which promoted sleep in the supine position, probably due to prior publicity of the need to put babies to sleep supine.

The major risk factors for sudden infant death
Parental smoking – antenatal and post natal
Prone sleeping position
Male sex
Maternal age (younger)
Low birth weight
Prematurity
Febrile illness
Thermal stress (high temperature, over wrapping)

The use of apnoea monitors has not reduced the risk of SIDS. There is no proven association of SIDS with the type of mattress used.

206. CHILD SEXUAL ABUSE   Answer: ABD

Child sexual abuse occurs when another person who is sexually mature involves the child in any activity which the other person expects to lead to their own sexual arousal. This includes exposure, pornography, sexual acts with the child and masturbation.

The prevalence suggested by a MORI poll in adults asking whether they had been abused as children (UK, 1985) is approximately 10%, this is probably an underestimate. 12% of females and 8% of males reported abuse.

About 60% of child sexual abuse is by an immediate family member. There is often a history of generational abuse.

There is a current conviction rate of abusers taken to court of 5%. The court cases are extremely distressing to the child, they may be accused of lying or feel that they have not been believed if conviction does not occur. The worry about not being believed is probably one reason for lack of disclosure in school age children who have been sexually abused.

Child sexual abusers often have a history of child sexual abuse (approximately 27% sexually abused as a child and 17% witnessed child sexual abuse) but this does not mean that all children who are abused go on to abuse.

Facts about abusers
31% fathers
4% mothers
10% older brothers
7% baby sitters
17% unrelated men (who may be part of an organised paedophile ring).

Anal fissures are common in children who are sexually abused. In children who are sexually abused there is an increased incidence of anorexia, headaches, recurrent abdominal pain, encopresis, enuresis and behavioural problems.

There is a higher prevalence of child sexual abuse in children with special educational needs.

Reflex anal dilatation is not a normal reflex. It may occur in inflammatory bowel disease, in chronic constipation, with the use of enemas and after anal stretch surgery, but it also occurs after anal penetration. The conclusion of the Cleveland Inquiry (1988) was that "...the sign of anal dilatation is abnormal and suspicious and requires further investigation. It is not in itself evidence of anal abuse."

Strong indicators of child sexual abuse are pregnancy, sexually transmitted disease, lacerations or scars in the hymen, anal fissures and positive forensic tests (semen).

Child sexual abuse is associated with physical abuse in 15% of cases.

207. PHYSICAL ABUSE IN CHILDREN   Answer: BCD

The reported incidence of physical abuse in children is 0.8/1000 (England and Wales 1983). It is characterised by a history inconsistent with the pattern of the injury.
- It is responsible for 200–300 non-accidental deaths per year in the UK.
- Mothers are more likely to be abusers than fathers.
- Handicapped children are at increased risk.
- It occurs in all social classes.

Risk factors include large family size, first born children (50%), low income, low parental intelligence, previous history of abuse in the parents and poor health of the parents (including alcohol and drug abuse).

The most common site of injury is the head and neck.

There may be abnormal coagulation in up to 16% of children in whom abuse is suspected.

Fractures are more common in pre school age children. Falls at home of 3–4 feet result in skull fractures of non-abused children in 1%. Complex and wide skull fractures are more common in abused children.

Intracranial injury is the commonest cause of death in abused children. 95% of serious head injuries in the first year of life are due to abuse. This is usually due to shaking injury which can lead to intracranial bleeding and is associated with retinal haemorrhages. The shaken child may also be hit against a hard object resulting in skull fracture and severe acceleration/deceleration injury.

Rib fractures are rarely seen in non-abused children. Periostial new bone formation is seen on X-ray 7–10 days after the initial injury.

208. SCHIZOPHRENIA   Answer: ACDE

Schizophrenia is characterised by particular abnormalities of thinking, perception and emotion. It is usually diagnosed between the age of 15–35 years, but the onset may be in childhood: early onset < 17 years, very early onset <13 years. The difficulty in diagnosing schizophrenia in childhood is that some symptoms are modified by the cognitive immaturity of the child and may not fit into the adult syndrome.

Symptoms include delusions, hallucinations, formal thought disorder (a disorder in the logic of thinking) and changes in affect. Immaturity of development particularly affects the severity of illogical thinking. Children with, or who go on to develop, schizophrenia may just seem odd.

The stages of schizophrenia are usually divided into an active phase where they are psychotic (lasts 1–6 months, shortened by anti-psychotic drug therapy), a recovery phase where there is a degree of impairment often with depression and a residual phase where recovery is incomplete (80%) leaving a degree of social and psychological impairment. It may progress to the chronic stage when a person may not recover from the acute stage.

Schizophrenia is uncommon in children, becoming more common after 15 years of age. Some of the difficulties in diagnosis in children may account for this. Whole life prevalence is 1%.

Family history is often positive. Lifetime incidence is 8% with an affected sibling, 12% if a parent is affected, 40% if both parents affected and 55% if an identical twin has schizophrenia.

The prognosis for recovery is 25–40% for adults, only a small minority recovering without further episodes. The prognosis is worse for early onset schizophrenia. The prognosis is better in females. There is a lifetime suicide risk of 15%.

209. SPEECH DELAY   Answer: BE

Recognised causes of speech delay include:
- Hearing defects
- Mental retardation due to any cause for example congenital hypothyroidism, tuberous sclerosis, Down's syndrome, Fragile X syndrome, intrauterine infections, and fetal alcohol syndrome
- Cerebral palsy

- Developmental expressive aphasia
- Emotional deprivation
- Autism

The family history is usually of relevance. There is often a history of speech delay in the parents, girls tend to speak earlier than boys, first born children tend to speak earlier than subsequent children and twins speak later than singletons. Tongue-tie, cleft palate and malocclusion may affect speech quality but do not cause speech delay.

Milestones in the development of speech
3–6 months
   Loud tuneful vocalisations
6–12 months
   Babbles in long repetitive syllables. Syllables 'da', 'ma' may be used from 8 months initially inappropriately but use in correct context to parents by 12–14 months.
1–1.5 years
   Starts using words in appropriate context. Understands many more words.
1.5–2.5 years
   Many intelligible words mixed with jargon. Starts asking 'why', 'where' questions by 2 years. Joins two or more words in phrases by 2 years.
2.5–4 years
   Period of rapid speech development with the acquisition of many new words. Constantly asking questions. Stops talking to him/herself during play in favour of directing speech towards others.
4+ years
   Can narrate stories, correct grammatical usage by 4.5 years.

Delay in any of these areas is a warning that there is a problem with either hearing or in speech acquisition.

210. DEVELOPMENTAL REGRESSION   Answer: CDE

This question distinguishes causes of developmental regression (the loss of previously acquired developmental milestones) from the causes of developmental delay (delay in acquisition of normal milestones).
It is useful to distinguish the age of onset of regression.

Regression before age of 2 years
HIV encephalopathy
Aminoacidurias
Hypothyroidism
Lysosomal enzyme disorders e.g. mucopolysaccharidoses, sphingolipidoses (e.g. Gaucher's disease), glycoprotein degradation disorders, mucolipidoses.
Mitochondrial disorders e.g. Leigh encephalopathy, Menkes kinky hair syndrome.
Neurocutaneous disorders e.g. neurofibromatosis, tuberous sclerosis
Genetic disorders of white and grey matter
Progressive hydrocephalus

Regression after 2 years of age
Subacute sclerosing panencephalitis
Late onset
Lysosomal enzyme disorders
Mitochondrial disorders
Genetic disorders of white and grey matter

211. NORMAL DEVELOPMENT   **Answer: ABE**

212. NORMAL DEVELOPMENT   **Answer: ABCD**

213. NORMAL DEVELOPMENT   **Answer: BCDE**

214. NORMAL DEVELOPMENT   **Answer: ACDE**

Normal developmental milestones
The reader is referred to a standard text book of development (see bibliography). Some useful milestones are:
4–6 weeks
 Smiles
6 weeks
 Prone-pelvis flat. Ventral suspension-head up to plane of body momentarily. Fixes and follows in the horizontal plane.
12–16 weeks
 Prone supports on forearms. Fixes and follows in the horizontal and vertical plane.
20 weeks
 Full head control. No head lag when pulled to sit. Reaches for objects and grabs them.

6 months
> Prone weight bears on hands. Rolls prone to supine. Transfers hand to hand. Chews. Feeds with a biscuit.

7 months
> Rolls supine to prone. Sits hands held forwards for support.

9 months
> Finger thumb opposition. Sitting can lean forward and recover position. Waves bye-bye. Starting to stand with support from furniture.

1 year
> Walking with one hand held. Uses two words with meaning. Mouthing stops.

13 months
> Stands alone for a moment.

18 months
> Goes up and down stairs holding rail. Can throw a ball without falling. Domestic mimicry. Feeds with spoon. Spontaneous scribble. Takes off socks and shoes. Can follow simple orders. Uses many words, jargon still present. Tower of 3–4 cubes. Dry in day.

2 years
> Goes up and down stairs two feet per step. Kicks ball without falling. Washes and dries hands. Tower of 6–7 cubes. Puts on socks, pants and shoes. Imitates vertical stroke. Turns pages one at a time. Joins two words in sentences.

2.5 years
> Jumps with both feet. Walks on tiptoes. Pencil held in hand not in fist. Knows sex and full name. Names one colour.

3 years
> Upstairs one foot per step, downstairs two feet per step. Rides tricycle. Attends to toilet needs without help. Dresses and undresses if helped with buttons and shoes. Names two colours. Constantly asks questions. Copies a circle.

4 years
> Up and downstairs one foot per step. Buttons clothes fully. Catches a ball. Copies a cross. Names three colours. Speech is grammatically correct and can give age. Eats with spoon and fork. Brushes teeth. Understands taking turns and sharing. Distinguishes past, present and future and right and left. Can hop for a few seconds on each foot.

5 years
> Can skip and hop. Drawing skills are improved – draws square (4.5 years) and triangle (5.5 years), can write a few letters. Names four colours. Can give home address. Distinguishes morning from

afternoon. Dresses and undresses alone. Chooses own friends. Understands needs for rules in games and play.

215. TOE WALKING   Answer: ABCE

Toe walking is common between ages 1 and 2. In most cases it is a habit and these children can stand on their heels without difficulty and ankle movements are normal.

Other causes
Prematurity
Spastic cerebral palsy
Congenital shortening of the achilles tendon
Duchenne muscular dystrophy
Peroneal muscular atrophy
Infantile autism
Spinal tumour
Unilateral hip dislocation

216. GUILLAIN-BARRE SYNDROME   Answer: ABC

The pathology of Guillain-Barre syndrome is inflammation with segmental demyelination in peripheral nerves. It is commonly preceded by an upper respiratory tract infection (10–14 days) and can follow gastroenteritis.

Implicated infectious agents
Epstein-Barr virus
Coxsackie virus
Influenza virus
ECHO virus
Cytomegalovirus
Mycoplasma pneumoniae
Campylobacter

The initial symptoms are of numbness and paraesthesia followed by progressive weakness. This generally starts in the lower limbs and 'ascends' over days or weeks. Weakness is usually symmetrical (90%). Power and tone are reduced with absent or reduced reflexes. About 50% have bulbar involvement. Myalgia may occur early in the disease.

Autonomic involvement can occur with flushing and hypotension. Bladder dysfunction may occur early in the disease in about 20%. 50% have cranial nerve involvement.

CSF protein rises with a normal CSF white cell count and glucose.

Close monitoring of the vital capacity is essential. Type II respiratory failure can occur secondary to muscle weakness.

Recovery is usually complete and treatment largely supportive. Relapses can occur in up to 5% of children. Plasmapheresis, intravenous immunoglobin, steroids and immunosuppressive drugs are used in patients with rapidly progressive ascending paralysis.

217. SPINAL MUSCULAR ATROPHY (SMA)   Answers: AB
(ANTERIOR HORN CELL DISEASE)

Three types
- Acute infantile spinal muscular atrophy, SMA type I, Werdnig-Hoffmann disease.
- Intermediate Spinal Muscular Atrophy (late infantile), SMA type II, chronic Werdnig-Hoffmann disease.
- Juvenile spinal muscular atrophy – which is Kugelberg–Welander disease.

All three are usually inherited in an autosomal recessive manner. The gene locus for all three types is on chromosome 5 and they are all variants of the same disease. The age of presentation varies with each disorder. SMA type I presents between 0 and 6 months, SMA type II between 3 and 15 years and Kugelberg–Welander between 5 and 15 years. Survival of SMA type I is rare beyond 3 years.

Clinical features
Hypotonia
Weakness
Absent reflexes
Fasciculation of the relaxed tongue
Normal intelligence

Diagnosis
DNA studies
CPK raised but can be normal
EMG – fibrillation potentials
Muscle biopsy – characteristic

Differential diagnosis of Kugelberg–Welander disease
Duchenne muscular dystrophy
Fascioscapulohumeral muscular dystrophy
Limb girdle dystrophy
Inflammatory myopathies

218. EPILEPSY   Answer: AC

Simple and complex differentiates between seizures in which consciousness is retained (simple) and those in which consciousness is impaired or lost (complex).

Partial seizures begin focally. They can become generalised (secondary generalisation).

Symptomatic epilepsy is when the cause is known. Cryptogenic is when there is a likely but unidentified cause and idiopathic is when no cause is known. Most childhood epilepsy is idiopathic.

An aura is not necessary for the diagnosis of childhood epilepsy.

219. TUBEROUS SCLEROSIS   Answer: ABCD

This shows an autosomal dominant inheritance with a 50% recurrence risk in offspring. 70% are new mutations. The prevalence in children is 1 in 10 000–15 000. The gene is on chromosomes 9 and 11.

Seizures are common, often presenting as infantile spasms. All seizure types except petit mal have been described in tuberous sclerosis. Tuberous sclerosis is a cause of symptomatic epilepsy. The age of seizure onset and the severity of mental handicap are directly related, with most children in whom seizures develop under the age of two suffering mental handicap. Seizures respond well to anticonvulsants but rarely with complete seizure control. Vigabatrin is indicated particularly in seizures associated with hypsarrythmia on the EEG.

Prevalence of mental handicap is 30–50%.

Clinical features

Skin	Hypopigmented macules
	Adenoma sebaceum present in 85% over the age of 5 years
	Periungual fibromas
	Shagreen patches
	Café au lait spots
Teeth	Enamel hypoplasia
Eyes	Choroidal hamartomas
CNS	Cerebral astrocytoma, malignant glioma, hydrocephalus
Kidney	Renal angiomas and polycystic kidneys
Cardiac	Rhabdomyomas
GI	Rectal polyp

Investigation
Echocardiography
SXR
EEG
CT
MRI

Early death may occur due to seizures or tumours affecting the CNS, heart or kidney.

Causes of calcification on skull X-ray
Arteriovenous malformation
Tuberous sclerosis
Sturge-Weber syndrome
Toxoplasmosis
Cytomegalovirus infection
Glioma
Astrocytoma
Craniopharyngioma

220. CEREBRAL PALSY   Answer: ABC

Cerebral palsy is the commonest cause of severe neurological disability in childhood. It is a disorder of posture and movement that results from a static injury to the developing brain. Although the injury is static the manifestations will change as the child develops and diagnosis is not always clear until late infancy. About 20% have mental retardation.

Prevalence
Prevalence is 2–4 per 1000 live births. Male to female ratio is 1.5:1.

Aetiology
Idiopathic (75%)
Known aetiologies are divided into pre, peri or post natal onset. These include hypoxia, infection, trauma, genetic and cerebral malformation. There is a strong association with low birth weight (51 per 1000 live births under 1500 g will have cerebral palsy), but these only account for a small amount of the total number of children with cerebral palsy. Perinatal asphyxia accounts for no more than 8%.

Classification

There are several different classifications of cerebral palsy. The Swedish classification is generally used:

- Diplegic
- Quadriplegic
- Hemiplegic
- Dyskinetic (athetoid)
- Ataxic

221. PETIT MAL EPILEPSY   Answer: DE

This accounts for 5% of childhood epilepsy. The peak age is 3–12 years. It is commoner in females. It shows an abnormal ictal EEG with 3 per second spike and generalised wave discharges. The inter-ictal EEG is normal. Hyperventilation will provoke seizures.

There is no known aetiology. Clinically, it is characterised by sudden cessation of speech and motor activity with a blank facial expression and flickering of the eyelids. There is no aura or post-ictal states. Tone is not lost but the head may fall forwards.

The drugs of choice are sodium valporate and ethosuximide. The long-term prognosis is good with most patients becoming seizure free by adolescence although a number do develop generalised seizures.

222. CEREBRAL PALSY   Answer: DE

Prenatal causes

Genetic forms – autosomal recessive and autosomal dominant
Cerebral malformation
Alcohol
Substance abuse
Infection (TORCH)
Intra-uterine growth retardation

Perinatal causes

Hypoxic ischaemic encephalopathy
Ventricular haemorrhage (preterm babies)

Postnatal causes
Meningitis
Encephalitis
Head injury

Preterm delivery is a risk factor for, but not a cause of, cerebral palsy.

223. INFANTILE SPASMS   Answer: ACDE

These represent 1–5% of childhood epilepsy. The incidence is 1–3 per 10,000 live births. It is more common in boys. Onset is usually between 4 and 9 months. The spasms are brief and transient but often occur in clusters. A spasm is due to a sudden muscular contraction which is usually generalised and a mixture of flexion and extension. Clusters of as many as 100 spasms can occur.

The EEG is characteristic and shows hypsarrhythmia (high voltage with multifocal spikes, spike and wave discharges, chaotic slowing and asynchrony). This is an inter-ictal appearance and may be suppressed during seizure activity. The EEG can be normal. The EEG is not of prognostic value in individual children.

Aetiology:
Symptomatic 70–80%
    Hypoxic-ischaemic encephalopathy
    Dysgenesis e.g. tuberous sclerosis, Sturge-Weber syndrome
    Infection pre, peri or post natal
    Haemorrhage intraventricular haemorrhage
    Metabolic e.g. neonatal hypoglycaemia
Idiopathic 20–30%

Traditional treatment is with high dose prednisolone or ACTH to which 70% have a good response. More recently vigabatrin has been used at doses of up to 200 mg/kg/day with good effect and a better safety profile. In many centres vigabatrin has now become the drug of first choice. Its effect is particularly good in seizures secondary to tuberous sclerosis.

Other drugs often used:
Nitrazepam
Sodium valproate
Lamotrigine

The prognosis is worse in the symptomatic group. Early recognition and early treatment of seizures is of benefit.
- 70% have severe developmental delay
- 50–60% develop chronic epilepsy which will be part of a chronic epilepsy syndrome
- 25–30% go on to develop the Lennox-Gastaut syndrome.

224. HYPOTONIA   Answer: BDE

Hypotonia in the infant can be as a result of neurological abnormality or systemic disease, and the differential diagnosis is wide. Infants implies less than 12 months and the age of presentation needs to be considered when the correct answers are selected. Becker's muscular dystrophy presents in late childhood (6–16 years) as does subacute sclerosing panencephalitis. The latter is more likely to manifest with hypertonia.

Neurological causes of hypotonia
Cerebral
    Encephalopathy
        e.g. birth asphyxia presenting as hypotonic cerebral palsy
    Normal brain structure
        Trisomy 21, Prader-Willi syndrome
        Hydrocephalus
        Agenesis of corpus callosum
    Degenerative disease e.g. metachromatic leukodystrophy
    Neurometabolic disease e.g. Zellweger's
Spinal Cord
    Transection e.g. following complicated breech delivery
    Spina bifida
Anterior horn cell disease
    Spinal muscular atrophy (Werdnig-Hoffmann's disease)
    Type II glycogen storage disease
    Poliomyelitis
Peripheral nerve disease
    Guillain-Barre syndrome
Disease of the myoneural junction
    Myasthenia gravis
Diseases of the muscle
    Congenital muscular dystrophy
    Congenital myotonic dystrophy

Systemic causes of hypotonia
Most acute and chronic childhood illnesses will cause hypotonia; particular examples include
- Hypercalcaemia
- Renal tubular acidosis
- Rickets
- Hypothyroidism
- Coeliac disease
- Cystic fibrosis
- Failure to thrive

225. CEREBRAL LESIONS   Answer: ADE

Features of a frontal lobe lesion
Disinhibition
Presence of the grasp reflex
Impaired memory

Abnormal micturition behaviour

The prefrontal lobe is concerned with aspects of psychological reactions, the ability to make intelligent anticipation of the future and the emotional consequence of thought.

Features of a precentral gyrus lesion
Pyramidal tract lesion (upper motor neurone lesion)
Contralateral hemiparesis

Features of a parietal lobe lesion
Spatial disorientation
Apraxia (loss of the ability to perform a pattern of movements although the purpose is known)
Agnosia (loss of the ability to recognise a previously familiar object)
Sensory inattention
Receptive dysphasia
Contralateral homonymous hemianopia (lower quadrant or both)

Features of an occipital lobe lesion
Flashing lights
Contralateral homonymous hemianopia

Features of a temporal lobe lesion
Visual sensations
Auditory/gustatory/olfactory hallucinations
Receptive dysphasia
Contralateral homonymous hemianopia (upper quadrant)

226. BENIGN ROLANDIC EPILEPSY   Answer: CD

This is commoner in boys with a peak incidence at age 2–14 years. It represents 15–20% of childhood epilepsy. It is often called benign partial epilepsy with centro-temporal spikes.

The fits are often preceded by an aura. The seizures themselves are short lived (1–2 minutes) and include paraesthesia and unilateral tonic-clonic convulsions involving the face, lips, tongue, pharyngeal and laryngeal muscles. Consciousness is usually preserved and seizures usually occur on wakening. Generalised (nocturnal) seizures often occur especially in children under the age of 5 years. There are a proportion of children with this syndrome who only have nocturnal seizures.

Inter-ictal EEGs often show centro-temporal spikes.

Carbamazepine is the drug of choice and fits are well controlled on it. In some children treatment is not required. Seizures generally disappear around puberty.

227. CRANIAL NERVES   Answer: ABD

Features of a third (oculomotor) nerve lesion
Complete ptosis
Diplopia
Downward and lateral gaze (unopposed lateral rectus and superior oblique muscles)
Pupil dilatation
Failure of the pupil to react to light or to accommodation

Features of a fourth (trochlear) nerve lesion
Diplopia
Failure of inferio-lateral gaze (failure of the superior oblique muscle)

Feature of a sixth (abducent) nerve lesion
Diplopia
Failure of lateral gaze

Features of Horner's syndrome
Partial ptosis
Pupil constriction
Anhydrosis
Enophthalmia
Heterochromia iridis
Normal direct and consensual reflex

Causes of ptosis
Congenital
Horner's syndrome
Oculomotor nerve palsy
Myasthenia gravis

228. ATAXIA   Answer: AE

Clinical features
Incoordination of voluntary movement
Abnormal speech – dysarthria
Occular incoordination – nystagmus
Hypotonia
Intention tremor

Aetiology of congenital ataxia
Cerebellar malformation
Dysgenesis of the cerebellar vermis e.g. Joubert's syndrome
Cystic malformation of the posterior fossa e.g. Dandy Walker syndrome
Perinatally acquired e.g. hypoxic ischaemic encephalopathy

Aetiology of acquired ataxia
Acute
    Infectious and post-infectious e.g. mycoplasma, chickenpox, measles
    Structural lesions e.g. tumours, hydrocephalus
    Toxic e.g. lead, phenytoin
    Metabolic disorders
    Vascular – basilar artery thrombosis
Intermittent
    Migraine
    Epilepsy
    Inherited recurrent ataxia (e.g. Hartnup disease)
Progressive
    Structural e.g. tumours

DNA repair abnormalities e.g. ataxia telangiectasia, xeroderma pigmentosa
Metabolic e.g. Wilson's disease, leucodystrophies, abetalipoprotein-aemia
Spinocerebellar degeneration, Frederich's ataxia

Friedrich's ataxia

This is a progressive ataxia with pyramidal tract dysfunction. Inheritance is usually autosomal recessive. The gene locus is known and is on chromosome 9. It usually presents before the fifteenth birthday with loss of position and vibration sense. Other features include absent tendon reflexes, extensor plantars, nystagmus, pes cavus, kyphoscoliosis, cardiac abnormalities (hypertrophic cardiomyopathy) and an increased risk of diabetes mellitus. Treatment is largely supportive. Death is usually secondary to cardiac complications.

Ataxia telangiectasia

This is an autosomal recessively inherited condition. The gene locus is known and is on chromosome 11. The ataxia usually presents in early childhood with characteristic telangiectasia. A third of these children develop malignancy. There is an increased risk of recurrent infection with a low IgA and IgG. The alphafetoprotein is usually raised. There is a 50–100 fold greater chance of developing lymphoreticular malignancy as well as brain tumours.

229. PATTERNS OF INHERITANCE   Answer: AE

This is an important question. Patterns of inheritance are easy to ask in multiple choice questions and should be known.

The inheritance of the conditions listed are as follows:

Tuberous sclerosis	Autosomal dominant
Ataxia telangiectasia	Autosomal recessive
Colour blindness	X linked recessive
Haemophilia A	X linked recessive
Myotonic dystrophy	Autosomal dominant

Genetic anticipation

Genetic anticipation refers to the situation by which successive generations are more severely affected by a particular disease process and at a younger age. Examples of this include
• Fragile X syndrome

- Myotonic dystrophy
- Huntingdon's chorea

230. DUCHENNE MUSCULAR DYSTROPHY   Answer: BE

The incidence is 1 in 3000 live born males. The inheritance is X linked recessive. The gene locus known and is at Xp21. A third of cases represent a new mutation. Females may be symptomatic as a consequence of the random inactivation of one of the X chromosomes.

Cases usually present between the ages of 3 and 5 with weakness and calf muscle hypertrophy. The reflexes disappear early in the disease apart from the ankle jerk which disappears late. Creatinine phosphokinase is usually raised at birth and high at diagnosis. Diagnosis is made by electro-myography and muscle biopsy both of which show typical features. In addition, DNA studies can be done looking for the dystrophin gene.

Complications arise from cardiac, respiratory and skeletal muscle involvement.

Becker's muscular dystrophy
This presents later than Duchenne muscular dystrophy. The gene defect is known and is at the same locus as Duchenne muscular dystrophy. Cardiac and respiratory muscle involvement is rare. The creatinine phosphokinase is high at diagnosis. EMG and muscle biopsy are helpful in establishing a diagnosis.

McLeod syndrome
This a benign non-progressive late onset myopathy in which the creatinine phosphokinase is usually mildly raised. It is X linked. Symptoms are usually mild. Splenomegaly is often seen.

231. FEBRILE CONVULSIONS   Answer: CE

Febrile convulsions occur in 3–4% of children. The age range is variably quoted but usually between 6 months and 5 years. Simple (75%) febrile convulsions last less than 15 minutes and are associated with a good prognosis. Complicated (25%) are either focal in origin or prolonged. These have a worse prognosis.

Risk factors for recurrent febrile seizures include previous febrile seizures and a positive family history of febrile seizures. The risk factor for siblings of an index case is 10% and the risk if either parent had febrile convulsions is 15%. There is no sex difference. There is no increased risk if there is a family history of epilepsy. A third of children who have a first fit will have a second and a third of these will have a third.

Risk factors for the development of epilepsy
Positive family history of epilepsy
Prolonged or atypical seizure
Pre-existing neurological problem
Abnormal neurological examination

Prophylactic anticonvulsants are not helpful in children with recurrent simple febrile seizures. The use of oral diazepam at the time of fever is controversial.

An inter-ictal EEG is usually normal and the investigation is unhelpful, except in children presenting with atypical febrile seizures.

232. COMPLEX PARTIAL SEIZURES   Answer: AD

Complex partial seizures originate as focal (partial) seizures usually in the fronto-temporal region. They can become generalised and consciousness is impaired.
The symptomatology is complex. Possibilities include:
• Transient blankness, staring or confusion
• Abrupt alteration of mental state in the form of time relationships and memory
• Déjà vu
• Semi-purposeful automatisms e.g. lip smacking, chewing, swallowing.

The EEG changes are characteristic with focal discharges from the fronto-temporal region. The drugs of choice are carbamazepine, vigabatrin and sodium valproate. There is often a past history of febrile convulsions. Surgery may be helpful in a number of children with resistant seizures.

233. MYOCLONUS   Answer: ABD

Myoclonus is a simple jerk-like movement that is not coordinated or suppressible. The jerks are usually flexor and occur at an extremity. If the legs are involved a child may be thrown to the ground. In childhood epilepsy myoclonic jerks can either present as the main seizure type (benign myoclonic epilepsy of infancy) or be one of several seizure types seen in an epilepsy syndrome.

West's syndrome
Infantile spasms
Mental handicap
Hypsarrhythmia on the EEG

Lennox-Gastaut syndrome
Extension of West's syndrome occurring between the ages of 1 and 5 years.
Atypical absences, myoclonic, tonic and atonic seizures
EEG shows slow spike and wave discharges
90% show moderate to severe mental handicap

Landau-Kleffner syndrome
This is rare and is characterised by the near complete or complete loss of previously acquired language before the onset of seizures which develop in 70–80%. The EEG is usually abnormal and the outlook poor. Myoclonic jerks are not usually seen.

Janz syndrome
This is juvenile myoclonic epilepsy and is characterised by myoclonic episodes with preserved consciousness. The episodes often occur on wakening or following sleep deprivation. EEG abnormalities are usually seen and the response to sodium valproate is good. Prolonged treatment is required.

234. PERIPHERAL NERVE INJURIES   Answer: CE

Peripheral nerve injuries need to be revised as they are often the subject of questions.

The small muscles of the hand are supplied by the median and ulnar nerves.

The radial nerve (C5 to C8) supplies two muscle groups
- those that supinate the forearm
- the extensors of the fingers, wrist and elbow.
It also supplies sensation to the back of the hand. Injuries to the radial

nerve occur either at the axilla or the elbow. Injury at the axilla will result in an inability to extend the elbow and wrist drop. Involvement at the elbow will result only in wrist drop.

Klumpke's paralysis results from an injury to the lower part of the brachial plexus (C8 to T1). Clinically this manifests as a claw hand with failure of forearm flexion.

235. PRIMITIVE REFLEXES   Answer: BC

The Moro reflex
This is initiated by sudden movement of the neck and consists of a rapid abduction and extension of the arms with opening of the hands. Eliciting it helps to assess muscle tone. It usually disappears by 3 months. A decrease in it on one side may be an early sign of a hemiparesis.

The startle reflex
This is similar to the Moro reflex, but is elicited by a loud noise. There is no opening of the hands.

The grasp reflex
Stimulation of the palm causes it to close. This reflex usually disappears by 3 months.

The asymmetric tonic neck reflex
When a baby lies with its head to one side, the arm and leg are extended to the same side, and the arm and leg on the contralateral side are flexed, appears by 2–3 weeks and disappears by 3 months. Its persistence is suggestive of cerebral palsy.

The parachute reflex
This appears between 6 and 9 months and persists. It is elicited by holding the infant in ventral suspension and suddenly lowering him. The arms extend as a defence reaction. Asymmetry may be a sign of hemiparesis.

The Babinski (extensor plantar) response is normal up until about one year of age.

236. HYDROCEPHALUS   Answer: BCD

Macrocephaly is defined as a head circumference larger then 2 standard deviations from the normal age corrected mean. Normal/familial large head is the commonest cause of macrocephaly. Other causes are hydrocephalus, megalencephaly (large brain) and a thickened skull.

Hydrocephalus occurs due to an excess volume of cerebrospinal fluid in the skull vault. This can result from either increased production or impaired reabsorption and circulation.

Cerebrospinal fluid is formed in the choroid plexus principally within the lateral ventricle. It flows from the lateral ventricles through the foramen of Munro into the third ventricle and from there via the aqueduct of Sylvius into the fourth ventricle. It exits the fourth ventricle via the foramina of Lushka and Magendie for reabsorption principally through the arachnoid villi.

Hydrocephalus can be either communicating or non-communicating. Non-communicating occurs as a consequence of obstruction at some point in the ventricular system.

Megalencephaly is enlargement of the brain substance. Hydrancephaly refers to the replacement of the brain substance by cerebrospinal fluid.

Causes of communicating hydrocephalus
Meningitis
Post haemorrhagic
Choroid plexus papilloma
Meningeal malignancy

Causes of non-communicating hydrocephalus
Aqueduct stenosis
Arnold-Chiari malformation
Dandy Walker syndrome
Klippel-Feil syndrome
Mass lesion
Warburg's syndrome

Causes of megalencephaly
Genetic
Sotos syndrome
Achondroplasia
Incontinentia pigmentii
Neurofibromatosis
Tuberous sclerosis

Alexander disease
Canavan disease
Galactosaemia
Mucopolysaccharidosis

Causes of macrocephaly due to a thickened skull
Anaemia
Rickets
Renal dwarfism
Hyperphosphataemia
Osteogenesis imperfecta

237. MICROCEPHALY   Answer: ABCD

Microcephaly refers to a small head due to a small brain, the head circumference being less than 2 standard deviations below the mean when corrected for age and sex. There are other causes of a small head including craniosynostoses (premature suture fusion). Microcephaly can be primary or secondary. Primary microcephaly refers to the situation whereby there is a genetic or chromosomal abnormality that causes the brain to be small. Secondary microcephaly refers to the situation whereby the brain was initially normal but because of a disease process subsequent growth has been impaired.

Causes of primary microcephaly
Familial-autosomal dominant or autosomal recessive
Chromosomal/syndromes
    Trisomy 13,18 and 21
    Cri du chat
    Cornelia de Lange
Holoprosencephaly

Causes of secondary microcephaly
Intrauterine infection
Drugs
Placental insufficiency/alcohol/drugs
Hypoxic ischaemic encephalopathy
Meningitis/encephalitis

238. BRAIN TUMOURS   Answer: AB

Primary brain tumours are the second most common malignancy in childhood after leukaemia. Metastatic tumours are rare in childhood.

Between the ages of 2 and 12 years infratentorial (posterior fossa) tumours are the most common. Under the age of two and in adolescence supra and infratentorial tumours occur with the same frequency.

Tumours within the posterior fossa produce symptoms and signs of raised intracranial pressure. Supratentorial tumours produce focal signs dependent on the tumour site. Personality changes can occur as a consequence of either.

Infratentorial (posterior fossa) tumours
Medulloblastoma – commonest brain tumour in children under the age of 7 years
Brain stem glioma
Ependymoma
Astrocytoma

Supratentorial tumours
Craniopharyngioma – common, present with bitemporal visual field defect, treatment is surgical and radiotherapy, residual hypothalamo-pituitary problems are common
Optic glioma
Pineal tumour
Oligodendroglioma

239. NEUROFIBROMATOSIS   Answer C

Eight types have been described at the time of writing. Types one and two are the most common.

Type one
- 1 in 4000
- 90% of all cases of neurofibromatosis
- autosomal dominant inheritance
- 50% new mutations
- gene locus on chromosome 17

Diagnosis of type one
If two of the following features are present:
- Axillary or inguinal freckling
- Optic gliomas (15%)
- Distinctive osseous lesion e.g. kyphoscoliosis, tibial bowing
- Two or more neurofibromas or one plexiform neurofibroma

- Two or more Lisch (iris) nodules (90%, do not occur in type two)
- Prepubertal child 5 or more café au lait spots greater than 5 mm diameter
- Post pubertal 6 or more café au lait spots greater than 15 mm diameter
- A first degree relative with neurofibromatosis

Café au lait spots are usually present at birth.

Less than 10% of patients are mentally retarded.

There are many other clinical manifestations and these should be reviewed.

Maternal folate deficiency is a risk factor for spina bifida.

There is an increased incidence of the following in type one neurofibromatosis:
- Phaeochromocytoma
- Rhabdomyosarcoma
- Leukaemia
- Will's tumour
- Seizures
- Neurofibrosarcoma
- Schwannoma

Conditions associated with café au lait spots
Neurofibromatosis
Tuberous sclerosis
Ataxia telangiectasia
Fanconi's anaemia
McCune Albright syndrome
Russell Silver dwarfism
Bloom syndrome
Gaucher disease
Chediak-Higashi syndrome
Normal variant

Type two
- Represents 10% of all cases of neurofibromatosis
- Autosomal dominant inheritance
- Mostly new mutations
- Gene locus on chromosome 22

Diagnosis of type two

Bilateral acoustic neuromas

or

Unilateral acoustic neuroma and first degree relative with neuro-fibromatosis type two

or

Two of the following – neurofibroma, meningioma, glioma, schwanoma, juvenile posterior subscapular lenticular opacities

240. BELL'S PALSY   Answer: ABDE

This is an acute unilateral facial palsy (lower motor neurone lesion). It usually occurs 2 weeks after a viral infection. Implicated agents include
*   Epstein Barr virus
*   Herpes virus
*   Mumps

Other aetiologies include hypertension.

Prognosis is excellent with a full recovery in more than 85% and permanent weakness in around 5%. Steroids are not proven to be helpful although often prescribed.

Other causes of facial nerve palsy

Tumour invasion

Trauma

Birth injury

Other causes of facial weakness

Myotonic dystrophy

Fascioscapulohumeral muscular dystrophy

Myasthenia gravis

BIBLIOGRAPHY

General
DP Addy, *Investigations in Paediatrics*, Saunders 1994
RE Behrman et al, *Nelson Textbook of Paediatrics*, 15th edition, WB Saunders 1995
GS Clayden et al, *Treatment and Prognosis: Paediatrics*, Heinemann Medical Books 1988
AGM Campbell et al, *Forfar and Arneil's Textbook of Paediatrics*, 4th edition, Churchill Livingstone 1992
AEM Davies et al, *Key Topics in Paediatrics*, Bios Scientific Publishers 1994
JA Eyre et al, *Paediatric Speciality Practice for the 1990s*, Royal College of Physicians of London 1991
FA Oski et al, *Principles and Practice of Paediatrics*, 2nd edition, Lippincott 1994

Child Abuse
CJ Hobbs et al, *Child Abuse and Neglect : A Clinician's Handbook*, Churchill Livingstone 1993

Community Paediatrics and Child Development
RS Illingworth, *The Normal Child*, 10th edition, Churchill Livingstone 1991
L Polnay et al, *Community Paediatrics*, 2nd edition, Churchill Livingstone 1993

Emergencies
K Mackway-Jones et al, *Advanced Paediatric Life Support: The Practical Approach*, 2nd edition, Advanced Life Support Group, British Medical Association 1997

Endocrinology
CGD Brook, *A Guide to the Practice of Paediatric Endocrinology*, Cambridge University Press 1993

Infectious Disease
EG Davies et al, *Manual of Childhood Infections*, British Paediatric Association, WB Saunders 1996

Immunisation
Department of Health, *Immunisation Against Infectious Disease*, HMSO 1996

Bibliography

Neonatology
NRC Robertson, *A Manual of Neonatal Intensive Care*, 3rd edition, Edward Arnold 1993

Nephrology
RJ Postlethwaite, *Clinical Paediatric Nephrology*, 2nd edition, Butterworth-Heinemann 1994

Neurology
R Appleton et al, *Epilepsy in Childhood and Adolescence*, Martin Dunitz 1995

Psychiatry
ME Garralda, *Managing Children with Psychiatric Problems*, British Medical Association 1993

Respiratory
R Dinwiddie, *The Diagnosis and Management of Paediatric Respiratory Disease*, 2nd edition Churchill Livingstone 1997

INDEX